Clinical Trial Design Challenges in Mood Disorders

Clinical Trial Design Challenges in Mood Disorders

Edited by

Mauricio Tohen
University of New Mexico Health Sciences Center
Albuquerque, NM, USA

Charles L. Bowden
University of Texas Health Science Center at San Antonio
San Antonio, TX, USA

Andrew A. Nierenberg
Massachusetts General Hospital; Harvard Medical School
Boston, MA, USA

John R. Geddes
University of Oxford, Oxford, UK

AMSTERDAM • BOSTON • HEIDELBERG • LONDON
NEW YORK • OXFORD • PARIS • SAN DIEGO
SAN FRANCISCO • SINGAPORE • SYDNEY • TOKYO

Academic Press is an imprint of Elsevier

Academic Press is an imprint of Elsevier
32 Jamestown Road, London NW1 7BY, UK
525 B Street, Suite 1800, San Diego, CA 92101-4495, USA
225 Wyman Street, Waltham, MA 02451, USA
The Boulevard, Langford Lane, Kidlington, Oxford OX5 1GB, UK

Notices
Knowledge and best practice in this field are constantly changing. As new research
and experience broaden our understanding, changes in research methods, professional
practices, or medical treatment may become necessary.

Practitioners and researchers must always rely on their own experience and knowledge
in evaluating and using any information, methods, compounds, or experiments
described herein. In using such information or methods they should be mindful of their
own safety and the safety of others, including parties for whom they have a professional
responsibility.

To the fullest extent of the law, neither the Publisher nor the authors, contributors, or
editors, assume any liability for any injury and/or damage to persons or property as a
matter of products liability, negligence or otherwise, or from any use or operation of
any methods, products, instructions, or ideas contained in the material herein.

British Library Cataloguing-in-Publication Data
A catalogue record for this book is available from the British Library.

Library of Congress Cataloging-in-Publication Data
A catalog record for this book is available from the Library of Congress.

ISBN: 978-0-12-405170-6

For Information on all Academic Press publications
visit our website at http://store.elsevier.com/

Typeset by MPS Limited, Chennai, India
www.adi-mps.com

Printed and bound in the United States of America

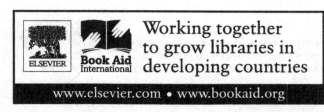

ELSEVIER Book Aid International Working together
to grow libraries in
developing countries

www.elsevier.com • www.bookaid.org

Contents

List of Contributors

Chittaranjan Andrade   National Institute of Mental Health and Neurosciences, Bangalore, India

Tim Appaiah   ClinPrax Research Pvt Ltd, Bangalore, India

Lesley Berk   Deakin University, School of Medicine, Geelong, VIC, Australia; The University of Melbourne, Parkville, VIC, Australia

Michael Berk   Centre for Youth Mental Health, Parkville, VIC, Australia; Deakin University, School of Medicine, Geelong, VIC, Australia; Florey Institute for Neuroscience and Mental Health, Parkville, VIC, Australia; The University of Melbourne, Parkville, VIC, Australia

Charles L. Bowden   University of Texas Health Science Center at San Antonio, San Antonio, TX, USA

Peijun Chen   Case Western Reserve University School of Medicine, Cleveland, OH, USA; Louis Stokes Cleveland VA Medical Center, Cleveland, OH, USA

Núria Cruz   University of Barcelona, Barcelona, Spain

Olivia Dean   Deakin University, School of Medicine, Geelong, VIC, Australia; The University of Melbourne, Parkville, VIC, Australia

Maurizio Fava   Harvard Medical School, Boston, MA, USA

John R. Geddes   University of Oxford, Oxford, UK

Heinz Grunze   Newcastle University, Newcastle-upon-Tyne, UK

Hong Jin Jeon   Harvard Medical School, Boston, MA, USA; Samsung Medical Center, Sungkyunkwan University School of Medicine, Seoul, Korea

Rasmus Wentzer Licht   Aalborg University Hospital, Aalborg, Denmark

Erin Michalak   University of British Columbia, Vancouver, BC, Canada

Andrew A. Nierenberg   Massachusetts General Hospital; Harvard Medical School, Boston, MA, USA

Willem A. Nolen   University of Groningen, Groningen, Netherlands

Renée Otmar   Deakin University, School of Medicine, Geelong, VIC, Australia

Martha Sajatovic   Case Western Reserve University School of Medicine, Cleveland, OH, USA

Vivek Singh University of Texas Health Science Center at San Antonio, San Antonio, TX, USA

Mauricio Tohen University of New Mexico Health Sciences Center, Albuquerque, NM, USA

Eduard Vieta University of Barcelona, Barcelona, Spain

Robert C. Young Weill Cornell Medical College, New York, NY, USA

Preface

Under the auspices of the International Society for Bipolar Disorders (ISBD), the editors enlisted the most experienced and creative minds in order to assemble a state-of-the-art book focused on the design of clinical trials in mood disorders with an emphasis on bipolar disorders. The task is timely. Since the late 1990s, a plethora of new designs and challenges have appeared that are addressed in this volume. To reach our goal, we mobilized a stellar group of contributors with academic, industry, or regulatory experience.

The scope of our audience is global. This is reflected in the geographical representation of our contributing authors who are from four different continents including North America, Europe, Asia, and Oceania. We have covered traditional designs and have included chapters on novel analytic techniques that have emerged in the second decade of the 20th century. In addition, we discuss a review of symptoms rating scales and models alternative to the traditional efficacy clinical trial, such as effectiveness and 'smart' designs. We include a chapter on challenges in conducting studies in developing countries to round out our efforts.

Our audience is intended to be individuals working on treatment studies on depressive and bipolar disorders including physicians, other behavioral health investigators, and quantitative scientists who are employed in academia, government, regulatory agencies, or the pharmaceutical industry. Our ultimate goal is to improve the lives of those people who have depressive and bipolar disorders. By improving the design and analytic techniques of studies, we hope to obtain valid, precise, and reliable answers about what works better and faster for our patients. Our vision is to collaborate globally in developing new technologies, but to act locally in the application of our strategies to benefit the patients in our respective communities.

Mauricio Tohen
Albuquerque, New Mexico, USA
Charles L. Bowden
San Antonio, Texas, USA
Andrew A. Nierenberg
Boston, Massachusetts, USA
John R. Geddes
Oxford, UK

Chapter One

Clinical Trial Design of Maintenance Treatments in Bipolar Disorder

Mauricio Tohen

University of New Mexico Health Sciences Center, Albuquerque, NM, USA

CHAPTER OUTLINE

INTRODUCTION

The first well-controlled maintenance study in bipolar disorder was published in the early 1970s (Prien, Klett & Caffey, 1973). However, no controlled studies were published for the remainder of the century. It was not until 2000 that Bowden, Calabrese & McElroy (2000) published their results comparing valproate, lithium, and placebo. However, the design of maintenance studies in bipolar disorder gained major interest in recent years due to the availability of new

1

Clinical Trial Design Challenges in Mood Disorders. DOI: http://dx.doi.org/10.1016/B978-0-12-405170-6.00001-4

molecules. During the early 2000s, several placebo-controlled studies were published, including the placebo-controlled comparison of lamotrigine versus lithium (Bowden *et al.*, 2003; Calabrese *et al.*, 2003). Soon after, maintenance studies with atypical antipsychotic agents were published starting with olanzapine (Tohen *et al.*, 2005, 2006), followed by studies on aripiprazole (Keck *et al.*, 2007), quetiapine (Suppes *et al.*, 2009), ziprasidone (Bowden *et al.*, 2010), and intramuscular long-lasting risperidone (Quiroz *et al.*, 2010). In this chapter, we will review the major challenges surrounding the design of randomized controlled maintenance trials in bipolar disorder.

Compared with the design of acute studies, maintenance studies have additional inherent complexities, including trial duration, definitions of outcome, type of previous episode, definition of an episode, etc. A major challenge in the interpretation of results across trials is that there have not been consistent definitions of course and outcome, which makes comparison across studies difficult to interpret.

DESIGN OF MAINTENANCE TREATMENT TRIALS IN BIPOLAR DISORDER

Need for a Uniform Nomenclature of Course and Outcome in Bipolar Disorders

Attempts have been made to develop a uniform definition of outcome.

Most recently, under the auspices of the International Society for Bipolar Disorders (ISBD), an international panel of experts proposed operational definitions in order to describe commonly used terms in clinical trials such as remission, recovery, relapse, and recurrence (Tohen, Frank & Bowden, 2009). The consensus panel also proposed definitions for other metrics commonly used in clinical trials and observational studies such as predominant polarity, switch, functional outcomes, and subsyndromal states. The use of consistent definitions is essential to improve patient care in order to make comparisons across studies. The task force acknowledged that the proposed definitions needed to be followed by further validation using existing databases and prospective use in observational studies and clinical trials. The task force suggested possible methodologies to validate the proposed operational definitions; for instance, the ability to predict duration of remission over a subsequent predetermined period could be used to validate response. Other validating techniques include the validation of symptoms severity scales such as the Montgomery and Äsberg Depression Rating Scale (MADRS) with cross-reference with an overall clinical global impression scale such as the Clinical Global Impressions (CGI) (Berk, Ng & Wang, 2008).

Clinical trials have been considered the gold standard for studying the efficacy and safety of pharmacologic treatments. By definition, a clinical trial is an experiment with patients as subjects of investigation (Rothman & Greenland, 1998). In general, the goal of a clinical trial is to evaluate the efficacy and safety of pharmacologic, device, or psychosocial treatments.

An ideal experiment would be designed by creating circumstances where all parameters on two contrasting populations remain stable with the exception of one factor affecting the outcome of interest. In the case of a maintenance treatment clinical trial comparing the difference of two maintenance treatments with the outcome time to a new episode in patients with bipolar disorder, the only variable that is different is the treatment to which patients are assigned through a randomization process (Rothman & Greenland, 1998; Tohen, 1992). Clinical trials represent the most valid tool to establish contrasts between two treatments. Their validity rest in three principles (Miettinen, 1985):

1. use of placebo or sham treatment to assure comparability of effects;
2. use of randomization to assure comparability of populations; and
3. use of blinding to assure comparability of information.

However, clinical trials may have limitations. First, inclusion and exclusion criteria need to be followed. The inclusion of some participants into clinical trials may not be ethical, for instance those with presence of suicidal thoughts or plans, thus limiting the generalizability of the findings. In addition, clinical trial findings may not be generalized if the protocol excluded participants whose condition was at a low risk of a particular outcome during a specified period of time. An example in bipolar disorder could be first-episode patients who had a low risk of relapsing in a short period of time or patients who were at a high risk of relapsing such as patients with a rapid cycling course. Other limitations include the lack of statistical power due to the combination of a small sample size and the selection of a rare outcome, such as relapse to a mixed episode, which would limit the possibility of finding a statistically significant treatment effect difference between treatments even when one does exist.

Trial Duration

In the design of clinical trials for maintenance treatment of bipolar disorder, one of the first questions faced by investigators is how long shall the duration of the trial be. A reasonable approach to the duration question is to take into account the clinical epidemiology of the condition, specifically what is the expected rate of relapses over a specified period of time. In order to differentiate prevention of relapses between two treatments, the duration of the observation time should be long enough to allow events (relapses) to take place. As mentioned above, epidemiologic data obtained from observational studies could be the basis of determining the length of a trial. For instance, Figure 1.1 shows a relapse survival curve of an observational study conducted at McLean Hospital, Belmont, MA (Tohen, Waternaux & Tsuang, 1990). As the curve depicts, 51% of patients had a relapse during the first year of follow-up. From year 1 to year 4, only an additional 23% of patients relapsed.

These findings can serve as the basis of making the decision of having a double-blind observation period of either 18 months (Tohen, Chengappa & Suppes, 2004) or 12 months (Bowden *et al.*, 2000, 2003; Calabrese *et al.*, 2003; Quiroz *et al.*, 2010; Tohen *et al.*, 2004, 2005, 2006). Other studies in

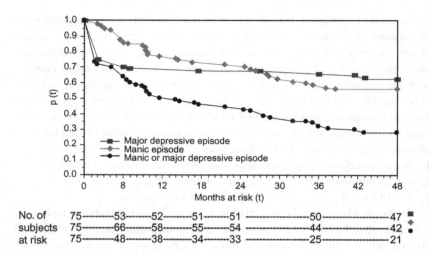

FIGURE 1.1 Cumulative probability of not relapsing. *Source: Tohen et al. (1990).*

maintenance treatments in bipolar disorder have utilized observation periods as short as 6 months (Bowden *et al.*, 2010; Keck *et al.*, 2007), which may limit the observation of events of interest. Of course, for other psychiatric or medical conditions, the observation period for a maintenance study should be determined by the clinical course of each condition.

An important consideration is that the expected time to relapse not only varies by individual but also within the same individual as the duration of time to new episodes will vary depending on the number of previous episodes in the same individual, which tends to be shorter as the number of episodes progresses but tends to plateau after the occurrence of three or more relapses (Goodwin & Jamison, 2007). It has also been suggested that the definition of relapse/recurrence should depend in the type of the index episode (Ghaemi, Pardo & Hsu, 2004; Goodwin & Jamison, 2007). The rationale is that if the natural course of manic episodes is expected to last 2–4 months and 3–6 months for depressive episodes then a differentiation should be specified in terms of the new episode being relapse to the same period episode or into a new episode (recurrence). In this case, the definition of relapse and recurrence would vary depending on the index episode. In other words, the duration of the remission period to consider recovery would vary depending on the type of the index episode where for index mania recovery would be defined as 8 weeks in remission while for depression recovery would require a longer duration. Therefore, if the goal is to prevent recurrence, then the duration definition would depend on the type of index episode. The ISBD task force based on the available empirical evidence did not support taking the type of index episode into account when differentiating re-emergence of the previous episode from emergence of a new episode. The key point to remember is that if these definitions help us in better understanding the natural course of the condition or the selective use of specific treatments, then its use is recommended but empirical evidence should back these definitions.

DEFINITION OF OUTCOME

Types of relapse or recurrence have been defined in different ways. Syndromal relapse has been defined utilizing Diagnostic and Statistical Manual of Mental Disorders (DSM) criteria (Tohen, Waternaux & Tsuang, 1990; Tohen *et al.*, 2003b, 2005, 2006). Other studies have use global rating scales (a four-point scale using the morbidity index (0 = no symptoms to 3 = hospitalization) or a six-point scale applied by clinicians (1 = no disturbance to 6 = extremely severe recurrence) (Greil *et al.*, 1997). In some clinical trials, symptomatic relapse has been widely used utilizing symptom rating scales, severity predetermined scores (Martinez-Aran *et al.*, 2008) (modified Rankin Scale (MRS) score > 16 or Depressive Symptoms Scale score > 25 (Bowden *et al.*, 2000), Young Mania Rating Scale (YMRS) score > 15 or Hamilton Depression Rating Scale (HAM-D) score > 15 (Tohen *et al.*, 2003a, 2005, 2006), or YMRS score > 20 or 24-item HAM-D score > 20 (Keck *et al.*, 2007; Quiroz *et al.*, 2010; Tohen *et al.*, 2005, 2006)). Other studies have defined outcome as the 'time to intervention', which can be needed to add a medication different to the active control, hospitalization, or withdraw from the study (Bowden *et al.*, 2000; 2003).

The definition of outcome is of major importance in a maintenance study as separation from comparators will vary depending on how 'new episodes' are defined. As mentioned before, authors have proposed differentiating relapse from recurrence depending on the duration of the remission period. The ISBD Consensus Panel defined relapse as when the new episode occurred in less than 8 weeks after remission was attained, which was defined as achieving recovery, and if the new episode occurred after recovery was achieved then recurrence would take place. Relapse was considered as re-emergence of symptoms of the same (index) episode, although it could be of the opposite pole, while recurrence was considered as the emergence of a separate episode.

Placebo-Controlled Maintenance Studies in Bipolar Disorder

The use of a placebo treatment group no doubt represents a challenge in recruiting participants but may also increase the potential of selection bias. Potential subjects of investigation are reluctant to take the risk of being assigned to placebo. Investigators are also equally concerned about who they enroll in a placebo-controlled trial. These concerns may lead to the enrollment of patients who have a history of low recurrences, which would lead to the recruitment of patients who may not recur even when assigned to placebo with the consequent loss of statistical power and generalizability of the results. As Baldessarini, Tohen and Tondo (2000) pointed out this may have been the reason why the placebo-controlled study led by Bowden *et al.* (2000) comparing valproate versus lithium was an unsuccessful study. The sample of the study included patients with mild severity scores with a history of low recurrences and close to 40% had never been hospitalized. In addition to limiting the generalizability of the results, another major concern was that the study appeared to lack the statistical power to detect a difference. We base this statement on the fact that studies have shown the best predictor of relapses is a history of multiple relapses (Tohen et al., 1990). In the Bowden et al. (2000) study, a population that had a history of moderate morbid history may have contributed to the low rate in the placebo arm. Importantly, the relapse rate of the lithium arm was similar to that of previous studies. An important contribution of the Bowden study was the importance of enriched designs in the selection of patients (Bowden et al., 1997). In this case, patients who during the acute phase responded to valproate were less likely to relapse if assigned to valproate compared with those patients who in the acute phase responded to a different treatment. This finding represents an example of an enriched design in the selection of patients for a maintenance study. Patients who in the acute phase respond to treatment 'A' were also likely to benefit from treatment 'A' during the prevention phase. Another type of enriched designed is to select patients who prior to randomization were exposed to the treatments being examined in order to assure tolerability (Bowden et al., 2003; Calabrese et al., 2003). It is essential that if two treatments are being compared, both treatments be enriched either for efficacy or tolerability such as the study comparing olanzapine versus lithium (Tohen et al., 2005) and the valproate versus lithium study (Bowden et al., 2000), where both drugs were given in the acute phase. Although enriched designs may limit the generalizability of the findings, in no way do they represent a biased result unless two treatments were being compared and only one of them was administered during the prerandomization phase. Furthermore, it also helps answer important clinical questions, that is if the treatment 'A' is effective and safe during the acute or premaintenance phase, is it also effective and tolerable during the prevention phase. Most relapse prevention studies in bipolar disorder that were designed in the early 2000s followed the enriched design (Bowden et al., 2003; Calabrese et al., 2003; Keck et al., 2007; Tohen et al., 2005, 2006).

Patient Recruitment

Diagnostic considerations, as well as severity of the condition, are important decisions in maintenance studies, as they will determine who enters the study and different aspects need to be considered as follows (Tohen, 2008).

COURSE OF ILLNESS

Considering that the risk of relapse increases with the number of previous episodes, inclusion criteria should specify the required minimum number of previous episodes. Considering that the natural course of the illness suggests that the median time between the first and the second episode is 4 years and also that there are patients who have had a single episode only (Tohen & Lin, 2006; Tohen et al., 1990), the exclusion of first-episode patients is reasonable.

Furthermore, at first episode, diagnoses may be unstable (Salvatore *et al.*, 2009). Some studies have required the presence of at least three previous episodes as the median time between the third and the fourth episode is 1 year. Some studies exclude patients with comorbid substance-use disorders (SUD), which has important implications in terms of generalizability of the results as the majority of patients with bipolar disorder have comorbid SUD. A challenge with including patients with comorbid SUD is an increase of nonadherence (Weiss *et al.*, 1998). In addition, SUD may be a confounder, thus it needs to be documented and controlled for in the statistical analysis. These issues need to be addressed in the analysis and interpretation of the results. A challenge to recruitment to efficacy studies is the need to discontinue current treatment (medication washout) and the majority of bipolar patients take three or more medications (Tohen *et al.*, 1990). Considering that discontinuation of psychotropic medications increases the risk of relapse (Faedda *et al.*, 1993; Suppes *et al.*, 1991, 1993; Viguera *et al.*, 1997), in order to minimize medication washout risks, investigators are likely to recruit patients with milder conditions, which may have an effect on study results.

Symptoms Ratings

Issues that need to be considered for the inclusion of patients are the accuracy of severity ratings to be considered in remission. Sachs *et al.* (2012) have proposed using computer-generated assessments to ensure the precision of the severity assessed. These techniques need to be considered in order to identify ineligible patients; however, the possible advantage of computer-generated rating over well-trained raters still needs to be determined. Advantages of computer-administered ratings may include consistency of metric across subjects of investigation and sites but they may also miss information only captured by trained clinician raters. Computer assessments no doubt may take care of rater bias but may also have an influence on the responses of subjects of investigation (Tohen, 2012). Other options include the use of central raters through teleconferencing. The goal is to improve the validity and reliability on the criteria that we use to determine patient eligibility into a study.

Statistical Considerations

Clinical trials published in the 21st century have uniformly utilized Kaplan Meier survival analysis methodology to estimate the efficacy of new molecules. Survival analysis provides estimates of time to a prespecified event such as relapse, treatment intervention, or study discontinuation. A concern with survival analysis is that it provides estimates to a single point in time. It provides only the quantity of how long it takes to reach an event but does not estimate what happens between randomization and reaching the outcome or extent to which patients are in full remission. Furthermore, it does not evaluate the quality of life during the time in remission. For bipolar disorder maintenance studies valuable information is lost if the patient's condition before reaching the specified outcome (relapse, intervention, or discontinuation) is not quantified. In the case of relapse, if it has been defined as reaching a prespecified score with a symptom rating scale, the period prior to relapse could include full remission of symptoms or presence of symptoms but with severity not reaching a relapse score. The latter state has been described as subsyndromal symptoms and was numerically defined by the ISBD Task Force (Tohen *et al.*, 2009). There is evidence that the presence of subsyndromal symptoms has implications both in terms of prediction of outcome (Tohen *et al.*, 1990; 2005), as well as in functioning (Marangell *et al.*, 2009). These limitations led investigators from the University of Texas Health Sciences Center at San Antonio, TX (Bowden *et al.* 2011; Tohen *et al.*, 2011) to explore novel ways of analyzing data in clinical trials (Tohen, 2007) and developed the Multi-state Outcome Analysis of Treatments (MOAT) methodology. Similar questions were faced by research in oncology where a method known as the Quality-adjusted Time Without Symptoms or Toxicity (QTWiST) was developed (Gelber *et al.*, 1995; Glasziou, Simes & Gelber, 1990). QTWiST has been applied in the analysis of chemotherapy oncology trials. The key component to QTWiST is to divide the survival or time at risk to an event divided into discrete periods that can be weighted by specific qualifiers such as tolerability, toxicity, or functioning. QTWiST methodology has proven to add value to the analysis of clinical trials in cancer research as it divides survival time into predefined periods such as survival with toxicity secondary to treatment that can have different degrees including survival without any toxicity. Patients, families, and caregivers can then give a different value to survival depending on quality of life providing 'quality-adjusted' survival times so additional survival times would have different values depending on the quality of life. MOAT was developed based on QTWiST methodology with adaptations specific to the condition. In the case of bipolar disorder, remission may mean absence of symptoms or presence of only mild symptoms. For example, prior to randomization, studies require a symptom rating score of less than a prespecified level. Most studies have utilized the YMRS (Keck *et al.*, 2007; Quiroz *et al.*, 2010; Tohen *et al.*, 2005, 2006) and have used a score of less than 12 to qualify as remission and 15 or more for relapse. During the follow-up period, patients have different degrees of severity.

The goal of MOAT is to measure a patient's condition across the observation time. No relapse time could be spent in full remission, subsyndromal mania, subsyndromal depression, subsyndromal mixed states, or full syndrome. Patients can also alternate from one state to another. MOAT adds up all periods for each state and determines if specific treatments influence the overall duration of the addition of all discrete periods for each state. In addition, weights could be assigned for side effects or tolerability. The program is available for download on the Internet (https://delta.uthscsa.edu/moat; last accessed 16 July 2014). The website provides recommendations for thresholds to establish clinical states and recommendations on common criteria for categorizing tolerability. Bowden and colleagues (2011) suggested that clinical states can be operationally defined as shown in Table 1.1.

Table 1.1 Clinical State Classification System (Seven Categories)

MRS	Hamilton Depression Scale – 17 Items	7–15	16+
0–5	Remission	SS depression	SYN depression
6–15	SS mania	SS mixed	SYN depression
16+	SYN mania	SYN mania	SYN mixed

MRS: modified Rankin Scale; SS: subsyndromal; SYN: syndromal.

Regulatory Considerations

Most clinical trials in maintenance study for bipolar disorders are funded by industry with the purpose of regulatory approval of maintenance treatment indication of new or existing compounds. Therefore, their design is very much determined by the expectation of regulatory agencies. Both the US Food and Drug Administration (FDA) and the European Medicines Evaluation Agency (EMEA) have made guidelines publically available. These guidelines have had a major impact in the design of clinical trials. In 2005, the FDA invited scientists from industry and academia to provide their perspective in the design of clinical trials in bipolar disorder (Psychopharmacologic Drugs Advisory Committee, 2005). The FDA requested input on issues pertaining to the design of maintenance trials in bipolar disorder. One key concern was the duration of the lead-in period. The position of the FDA was that this duration would provide the evidence of the specific length of the demonstrated duration. In other words, if the lead-in period was 1 week before randomization and the new treatment was statistically significant from a prespecified outcome such as time to relapse from the comparison or placebo treatment, then the study would provide evidence of maintenance efficacy not from the duration of the postrandomization period but rather from the lead in prerandomization period. The rationale was that instead of having a discontinuation study meaning time to relapse after a drug is discontinued, the lead-in period provided evidence that a compound was effective as once stopped the patient would relapse. A proposed lead-in period was a minimum of 3 months. This approach led to the change in lead-in periods from as short as 1 week in earlier studies (Tohen *et al.*, 2006) to 3 months in later studies (Keck *et al.*, 2007). Concerns about longer lead-in periods include the need for significantly larger samples as attrition prior to randomization increases with time. Other concerns include that it is not clear whether longer stabilization makes patients more stable or simply selects patients with a more stable course of illness. In addition, the interpretation of a 'negative' study would be difficult in the absence of a positive control. Furthermore, adding an active control would increase the sample size and time to completion further.

The EMEA and the Committee for Proprietary Medicinal Products (CPMP) have also published guidance on clinical investigations of molecules for the treatment and prevention of bipolar disorder (European Medicines Agency, 2001). The EMEA provided a definition of maintenance of effect as "the effect of treatment, seen in the short-term is maintained during the whole episode." Relapse was defined as "an increase in symptomatology immediately or almost immediately after medication is stopped"; and recurrence as "re-emergence of symptoms (new episode) after a time with no or minimal symptoms." Of note, the ISBD Task Force differentiated relapse from recurrence by the latter as a new episode following at least 8 weeks in remission (Tohen *et al.*, 2009). The EMEA position was that products could be approved for acute episodes and/or prevention of episodes (European Medicines Agency, 2001). Regarding study designs, the EMEA requires the inclusion of both active and placebo controls with lithium as a suggested comparator and with duration of at least 1 year.

CONCLUSIONS

The design of maintenance studies in bipolar disorder has evolved in recent years. Factors that have been considered include the selection of subject of investigation, the duration of the trials, and the use of a placebo. In addition, new statistical methodologies have been developed.

REFERENCES

Baldessarini, R., Tohen, M., & Tondo, L. (2000). Maintenance treatment in bipolar disorder. *Archives of General Psychiatry, 57*, 490–491.

Berk, M., Ng, F., Wang, W. V., et al. (2008). The empirical redefinition of the psychometric criteria for remission in bipolar disorder. *Journal of Affective Disorders, 106*, 153–158.

Bowden, C. L., Calabrese, J. R., McElroy, S. L., et al. (2000). For the divalproex maintenance study group: a randomized, placebo-controlled 12-month trial of divalproex and lithium in treatment of outpatients with bipolar I disorder. *Archives of General Psychiatry, 57*, 481–489.

Bowden, C. L., Calabrese, J. R., Sachs, G., et al. (2003). A placebo controlled 18-month trial of lamotrigine and lithium maintenance treatment in recently manic or hypomanic patients with bipolar I disorder. *Archives of General Psychiatry, 60*, 392–400.

Bowden, C.L., Mintz, J., & Tohen, M., et al. (2011). Development of novel integrative multistate measures of efficacy, tolerability and functional status in maintenance clinical trials for bipolar disorder. In: *Proceedings of the American College of Neuropsychopharmacology*; Dec 5 2011; Hollywood FL.

Bowden, C. L., Swann, A., Calabrese, J. R., et al. (1997). Maintenance clinical trials in bipolar disorder: design implications of the divalproex–lithium placebo study. *Psychopharmacology Bulletin, 33*, 693–699.

Bowden, C. L., Vieta, E., Ice, K. S., et al. (2010). Ziprasidone plus a mood stabilizer in subjects with bipolar I disorder: a 6-month, randomized, placebo-controlled, double-blind trial. *Journal of Clinical Psychiatry, 71*, 130–137.

Calabrese, J. R., Bowden, C. L., Sachs, G., et al. (2003). A placebo controlled 18-month trial of lamotrigine and lithium maintenance treatment in recently depressed patients with bipolar I disorder. *Journal of Clinical Psychiatry, 64*, 1013–1024.

European Medicines Agency. (2001). Note for guidance on clinical investigation of medical products in the treatment and prevention of bipolar disorder. <http://www.ema.europa.eu/docs/en_GB/document_library/Scientific_guideline/2009/09/WC500003528.pdf/> Accessed 16.07.14.

Faedda, G. L., Tondo, L., Baldessarini, R. J., et al. (1993). Outcome after rapid vs gradual discontinuation of lithium treatment in bipolar disorders. *Archives of General Psychiatry*, *50*, 448–455.

Gelber, R. D., Cole, B. F., Gelber, S., et al. (1995). Comparing treatments using quality-adjusted survival: the Q-TWiST method. *American Statistician*, *49*, 161–169.

Ghaemi, S. N., Pardo, T. B., & Hsu, D. J. (2004). Strategies for preventing the recurrence of bipolar disorder. *Journal of Clinical Psychiatry*, *65*(Suppl. 10), 16–23.

Glasziou, P. P., Simes, R. J., & Gelber, R. D. (1990). Quality adjusted survival analysis. *Statistics in Medicine*, *9*, 1259–1276.

Goodwin, F. K., & Jamison, K. R. (2007). *Manic-depressive illness: bipolar disorders and recurrent depression* (2nd ed.). New York: Oxford University.

Greil, W., Ludwig-Mayerhofer, W., Erazo, N., et al. (1997). Lithium versus carbamazepine in the maintenance treatment of bipolar disorders – a randomised study. *Journal of Affective Disorders*, *43*, 151–161.

Keck, P. E., Jr., Calabrese, J. R., McIntyre, R. S., et al. (2007). Aripiprazole monotherapy for maintenance therapy in bipolar I disorder: a 100-week, double-blind study versus placebo. *Journal of Clinical Psychiatry*, *68*, 1480–1491.

Marangell, L. B., Dennehy, E. B., Miyahara, S., et al. (2009). The functional impact of subsyndromal depressive symptoms in bipolar disorder: data from STEP-BD. *Journal of Affective Disorder*, *114*, 58–67.

Martinez-Aran, A., Vieta, E., Chengappa, K. N. R., et al. (2008). Reporting outcomes in clinical trials for bipolar disorder: a commentary and suggestions for change. *Bipolar Disorders*, *10*, 566–579.

Miettinen, O. (1985). *Theoretical epidemiology: principles of occurrence research in medicine*. Chichester: John Wiley & Sons.

Prien, R. F., Klett, C. J., & Caffey, E. M., Jr. (1973). Lithium carbonate and imipramine in prevention of affective episodes. A comparison in recurrent affective illness. *Archives in General Psychiatry*, *29*, 420–425.

Psychopharmacologic Drugs Advisory Committee. (2005). <http://www.fda.gov/oc/advisory/accalendar/2005/cder12544dd10252605.html/> Accessed 16.07.14.

Quiroz, J., Yatham, L., Palumbo, J., et al. (2010). Risperidone long-acting injectable monotherapy in the maintenance treatment of bipolar I disorder. *Biological Psychiatry*, *68*, 156–162.

Rothman, K. J., & Greenland, S. (1998). *Modern epidemiology* (2nd ed.). Philadelphia, PA: Lippincott-Raven Publishers.

Sachs, G., Vanderburg, D., Edman, S., et al. (2012). Adjunctive oral ziprasidone in patients with acute mania treated with lithium or divalproex: 2. Influence of protocol-specific eligibility criteria on signal detection. *Journal of Clinical Psychiatry*, *73*, 1420–1425.

Salvatore, P., Baldessarini, R. J., Tohen, M., et al. (2009). Two-year stability of DSM-IV diagnoses in 500 first-episode psychotic disorder patients. *Journal of Clinical Psychiatry*, *70*, 458–466.

Suppes, T., Baldessarini, R. J., Faedda, G. L., et al. (1991). Risk of recurrence following discontinuation of lithium treatment in bipolar disorder. *Archives of General Psychiatry*, *48*, 1082–1088.

Suppes, T., Baldessarini, R. J., Faedda, G. L., et al. (1993). Discontinuation of maintenance treatment in bipolar disorder: risks and implications. *Harvard Review of Psychiatry*, *1*, 131–144.

Suppes, T., Vieta, E., Liu, S., et al. (2009). Maintenance treatment for patients with bipolar I disorder: results from a North American study of quetiapine in combination with lithium or divalproex. *American Journal of Psychiatry*, *166*, 476–488.

Tohen, M. (1992). Bias and other methodological issues in follow-up (cohort) studies. In M. Fava & G. Rosenbaum (Eds.), *Research designs and methods in psychiatry* (pp. 119–125). Amsterdam: Elsevier.

Tohen, M. (2007). Collaborations between academic psychiatry and the pharmaceutical industry: a perspective from industry. *Epidemiologia e Psichiatria Sociale*, *16*, 197–198.

Tohen, M. (2008). Clinical trials in bipolar mania: implications in study design and drug development. *Archives in General Psychiatry, 65*, 252–253.

Tohen, M. (2012). Methodologies to avoid the enrollment of ineligible patients in clinical trials. *Journal of Clinical Psychiatry, 73*, 1426–1427.

Tohen, M., Calabrese, J. R., Sachs, G. S., et al. (2006). Randomized, placebo-controlled trial of olanzapine as maintenance therapy in patients with bipolar I disorder responding to acute treatment with olanzapine. *American Journal of Psychiatry, 163*, 247–256.

Tohen, M., Chengappa, K. N. R., Suppes, T., et al. (2004). Relapse prevention in bipolar I disorder: 18-month comparison of olanzapine plus mood stabiliser vs mood stabiliser alone. *British Journal of Psychiatry, 184*, 337–345.

Tohen, M., Frank, E., Bowden, C. L., et al. (2009). The International Society of Bipolar Disorders (ISBD) Task Force on the nomenclature of course and outcome of bipolar disorders bipolar disorders. *Bipolar Disorders, 11*, 453–473.

Tohen, M., Greil, W., Calabrese, J., et al. (2005). Olanzapine versus lithium in the maintenance treatment of bipolar disorder: a 12-month, randomized, double-blind, controlled clinical trial. *American Journal of Psychiatry, 162*, 1281–1290.

Tohen, M., Ketter, T. A., Zarate, C. A., et al. (2003a). Olanzapine versus divalproex sodium for the treatment of acute mania and maintenance of remission: a 47-week study. *American Journal of Psychiatry, 160*, 1263–1271.

Tohen, M., & Lin, D. (2006). Commentary on N. Ghaemi's "Hippocratic psychopharmacology of bipolar disorder" maintenance treatment in bipolar disorder. *Psychiatry (Edgmont), 3*, 43–45.

Tohen, M., Mintz, J., & Bowden, C.L., et al. (2011). Use of the functional adjusted clinical states in bipolar disorder methodology in the lamotrigine registration studies in bipolar disorder. In: *Proceedings of the american college of neuropsychopharmacology*; Dec 2–5 2011; Hollywood FL.

Tohen, M., Waternaux, C. M., Tsuang, M. T., et al. (1990). Outcome in mania. A 4-year prospective follow-up of 75 patients utilizing survival analysis. *Archives of General Psychiatry, 47*, 1106–1111.

Tohen, M., Zarate, C. A., Hennen, J., et al. (2003b). The McLean-Harvard First-Episode Mania Study: prediction of recovery and first recurrence. *American Journal of Psychiatry, 160*, 2099–2107.

Viguera, A. C., Baldessarini, R. J., Hegarty, J. D., et al. (1997). Clinical risk following abrupt and gradual withdrawal of maintenance neuroleptic treatment. *Archives of General Psychiatry, 54*, 49–55.

Weiss, R. D., Greenfield, S. F., Najavits, L. M., et al. (1998). Medication compliance among patients with bipolar disorder and substance use disorder. *Journal of Cliqnical Psychiatry, 59*, 172–174.

Chapter | Two

Meta-Analysis of Clinical Trials in Bipolar Disorder

John R. Geddes

University of Oxford, Oxford, UK

CHAPTER OUTLINE

INTRODUCTION

The methodology of reviewing has developed enormously over the since the mid-1980s. The key insight behind this rapid development was the recognition in the late 1980s that most scientists and clinicians rely on reviews of scientific evidence rather than primary studies for keeping up-to-date but that the methodology of reviews lagged behind developments of the methodology in primary research studies (Mulrow, 1987). Thus, it was demonstrated that recommendations tend to be based on biased samples of studies in which the selection of primary studies in the review was unsystematic, unreproducible, and often reflected the authors' existing ideas rather than producing an unbiased synthesis of the evidence. In one influential study, Antman and colleagues compared the recommendations of narrative conventional reviews with those of systematic reviews and demonstrated clearly that systematic reviews tend to be less positive about new interventions (Antman *et al.*, 1992). This finding was replicated in psychiatry (Cipriani & Geddes, 2003).

Clinical Trial Design Challenges in Mood Disorders. DOI: http://dx.doi.org/10.1016/B978-0-12-405170-6.00002-6

The recognition of the importance and poor quality of reviews led to several major initiatives. The Cochrane Collaboration (Chalmers & Haynes, 1994), an international collaboration dedicated to preparing, disseminating, and updating high-quality reviews of the effects of treatments, was founded. The methodology of systematic reviews was established with systematic reviews distinguished from non-systematic reviews by the presence of a specific methods section that described the search strategy, inclusion and exclusion criteria, and methods of data synthesis. The aim of systematic reviews was to identify an unbiased and comprehensive sample of primary studies that can then be summarized to produce a reliable estimate of the pooled treatment effect.

In those situations when the numeric results of the individual studies are compatible, it is possible to synthesize the quantitative results using the technique of meta-analysis. Numerical pooling of the results from multiple studies has two key benefits:

1. more precise estimates of the treatment effect are produced by the much larger sample sizes that result from the pooling of several trials and consequent reduction in random error;
2. investigation of variation, or heterogeneity, between the individual trials. There are many reasons why treatment effects may appear to vary between trials. However, first the variation might in fact be no more than expected by the play of chance alone and might not indicate true variation between studies. If there is more variation than can be explained by chance, then this might be because of clinical heterogeneity; in other words, there are differences in the treatment effect because there are differences between the patients, treatments, or comparisons.

REDUCTION OF RISK OF SUICIDE WITH LITHIUM: AN EXAMPLE OF INCREASED STATISTICAL POWER BY POOLING

One good example of the benefits of increasing statistical power is provided by the analysis of the potential reduction of risk of suicide in patients treated with lithium. Although observational evidence had suggested that lithium reduced the risk of suicide in patients with bipolar disorder (Tondo *et al.*, 1998), it was unclear whether or not this was a true effect of lithium or was due to confounding; in other words, it simply reflected the fact that patients who take lithium may be more compliant and less impulsive in general than patients who do not. Therefore, was the lower rate of suicide due to the lithium or other differences between the two groups of patients?

There are major, probably insuperable, difficulties in using a randomized trial design to detect a treatment effect on suicide. Although patients with bipolar disorder are at a lifetime risk of around 15% for suicide, the highest for any mental disorder, it is a very low event rate to study in a randomized trial. Achieving the sample size to be able to detect any benefit on suicide risk reliably is unlikely to be feasible.

However, by identifying all randomized trials that have compared lithium with placebo, it is possible to increase greatly the sample size. Cipriani *et al.* reported a meta-analysis of clinical trials investigating suicide risk and found that the risk of suicide was lower in patients treated with lithium than with placebo (Cipriani *et al.*, 2005). Although the result was statistically significant and would be of considerable clinical importance, the confidence interval around the estimate was wide due to the very low event rate. One updated meta-analysis published in 2013 reported an 87% reduction in the odds of suicide, and a 62% reduction in the odds of all-cause mortality in patients allocated to lithium compared with placebo (see Figure 2.1; Figure 2.2) (Cipriani *et al.*, 2013a).

Although this confidence interval around the treatment effect remains rather unstable and probably demonstrates the difficulty of investigating this outcome in randomized trials, the credibility of this treatment effect is enhanced by the fact that the treatment effect is very similar to that observed in observational studies that have much higher sample sizes and, therefore, event rates (Goodwin *et al.*, 2003). Another example of the identification of a treatment effect when individual studies have the problem of low power is the assessment of the effect of lamotrigine on bipolar depression. This review identified five randomized trials. Although no single trial found lithium to be

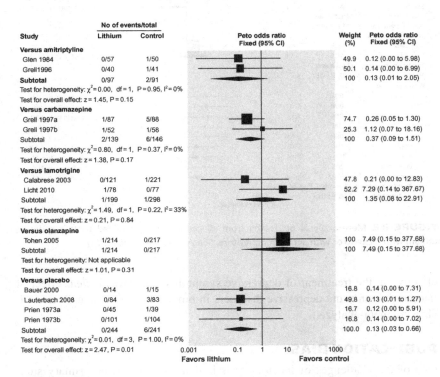

FIGURE 2.1 Meta-analysis of suicides in randomized trials comparing lithium with placebo or with active comparators. *Source: Cipriani et al. (2013).*

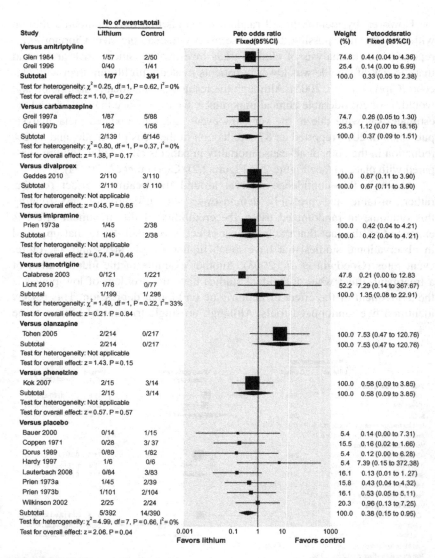

Study	No of events/total Lithium	Control	Peto odds ratio Fixed(95%CI)	Weight (%)	Petooddsratio Fixed (95%CI)
Versus amitriptyline					
Glen 1984	1/57	2/50		74.6	0.44 (0.04 to 4.36)
Greil 1996	0/40	1/41		25.4	0.14 (0.00 to 6.99)
Subtotal	1/97	3/91		100.0	0.33 (0.05 to 2.38)
Test for heterogeneity: χ^2=0.25, df=1, P=0.62, I^2=0%					
Test for overall effect: z=1.10, P=0.27					
Versus carbamazepine					
Greil 1997a	1/87	5/88		74.7	0.26 (0.05 to 1.30)
Greil 1997b	1/82	1/58		25.3	1.12 (0.07 to 18.16)
Subtotal	2/139	6/146		100.0	0.37 (0.09 to 1.51)
Test for heterogeneity: χ^2=0.80, df=1, P=0.37, I^2=0%					
Test for overall effect: z=1.38, P=0.17					
Versus divalproex					
Geddes 2010	2/110	3/110		100.0	0.67 (0.11 to 3.90)
Subtotal	2/110	3/110		100.0	0.67 (0.11 to 3.90)
Test for heterogeneity: Not applicable					
Test for overall effect: z=0.45. P=0.65					
Versus imipramine					
Prien 1973a	1/45	2/38		100.0	0.42 (0.04 to 4.21)
Subtotal	1/45	2/38		100.0	0.42 (0.04 to 4.21)
Test for heterogeneity: Not applicable					
Test for overall effect: z=0.74. P=0.46					
Versus lamotrigine					
Calabrese 2003	0/121	1/221		47.8	0.21 (0.00 to 12.83)
Licht 2010	1/78	0/77		52.2	7.29 (0.14 to 367.67)
Subtotal	1/199	1/298		100.0	1.35 (0.08 to 22.91)
Test for heterogeneity: χ^2=1.49, df=1, P=0.22, I^2=33%					
Test for overall effect: z=0.21. P=0.84					
Versus olanzapine					
Tohen 2005	2/214	0/217		100.0	7.53 (0.47 to 120.76)
Subtotal	2/214	0/217		100.0	7.53 (0.47 to 120.76)
Test for heterogeneity: Not applicable					
Test for overall effect: z=1.43. P=0.15					
Versus phenelzine					
Kok 2007	2/15	3/14		100.0	0.58 (0.09 to 3.85)
Subtotal	2/15	3/14		100.0	0.58 (0.09 to 3.85)
Test for heterogeneity: Not applicable					
Test for overall effect: z=0.57. P=0.57					
Versus placebo					
Bauer 2000	0/14	1/15		5.4	0.14 (0.00 to 7.31)
Coppen 1971	0/28	3/37		15.5	0.16 (0.02 to 1.66)
Dorus 1989	0/89	1/82		5.4	0.12 (0.00 to 6.28)
Hardy 1997	1/6	0/6		5.4	7.39 (0.15 to 372.38)
Lauterbach 2008	0/84	3/83		16.1	0.13 (0.01 to 1.27)
Prien 1973a	1/45	2/39		15.8	0.43 (0.04 to 4.32)
Prien 1973b	1/101	2/104		16.1	0.53 (0.05 to 5.11)
Wilkinson 2002	2/25	2/24		20.3	0.96 (0.13 to 7.25)
Subtotal	5/392	14/390		100.0	0.38 (0.15 to 0.95)
Test for heterogeneity: χ^2=4.99, df=7, P=0.66, I^2=0%					
Test for overall effect: z=2.06. P=0.04		0.001 0.1 1 10 1000			
		Favors lithium	Favors control		

FIGURE 2.2 Meta-analysis of deaths from all causes in randomized trials comparing lithium with placebo or with active comparators. *Source: Cipriani et al. (2013).*

effective in the treatment of depressive symptoms, there was a clear effect of lamotrigine on acute depressive disorders in bipolar disorder when all five trials were meta-analyzed.

PUBLICATION BIAS

One of the challenges of meta-analysis is that retrieval of the primary studies tends to select studies that have found a positive result. This is because these studies are more likely to be published in the first place, and published in higher impact, English language journals that are more likely to be included in bibliographic systems (Easterbrook *et al.*, 1991). The resulting publication bias is recognized as one of the most serious threats to the validity of meta-analysis. The presence and/or likelihood of publication bias can sometimes be inferred using techniques such as funnel plots (Gilbody *et al.*, 2000), but it remains a major problem when the systematic review relies on retrospective identification of the primary studies. Current attempts to minimize the effect of publication bias include calls to make prospective registration of all clinical trials mandatory (De Angelis *et al.*, 2004) and calls to make sponsors of trials (especially pharmaceutical companies) release all clinical trial data (see http://www.alltrials.net, last accessed 17 July 2014).

INDIVIDUAL PATIENT DATA META-ANALYSES

Even if an unbiased sample of primary studies is identified, a further challenge of meta-analysis is that the data have to be obtained from published reports that normally only contain aggregated or summary data. Key parameters such as standard deviations may not be reported and need to be imputed. Accessing the individual patient data (IPD) can transform the potential power of the meta-analysis because pooling can use a standardized approach across trials, which can reduce some of the variation in the results (Clarke & Stewart, 1994). Pooling the data increases power and subgroup analyses may be performed to investigate if the treatment effect is modified by particular patient or clinical characteristics. Unfortunately, it can be difficult to obtain IPD although more individual patient data meta-analyses (IPDMA) are appearing and the culture of data sharing will make them more feasible more frequently. There are few IPDMA in bipolar disorder; however, we were able to investigate the effect of lamotrigine in bipolar depression using IPD from all the trials conducted by GlaxoSmithKline (GSK) (Geddes *et al.*, 2008). Individual trials demonstrated no convincing treatment effect of lamotrigine compared with placebo but the overall pooled analysis found a small but statistical benefit. Use of IPD allowed investigation of the effect of baseline severity of symptoms on efficacy.

From Figure 2.3 it is clear that lamotrigine appears to be effective against depressive symptoms but more so when the baseline severity of depression is above 24 on the Hamilton Depression of Rating Scale. Although this may be thought to indicate an interaction of treatment effect by illness severity, in fact it is clear from the absolute response rates that this is probably explained by a higher placebo response rate in patients with a lower severity of illness because the placebo response rate is much higher in this group whereas the response rate on active medication remains approximately the same in both milder and more severely ill patients.

This variation in the effect of placebo could either represent the fact that patients who are more mildly ill are more likely to respond to placebo or it

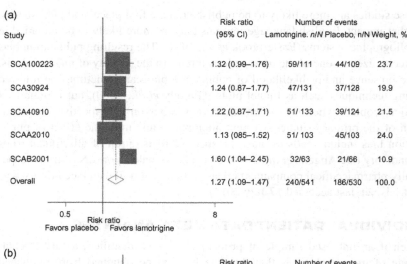

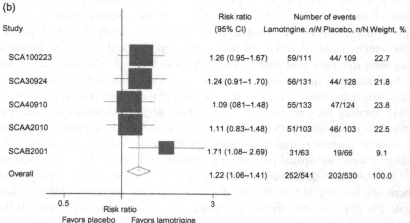

FIGURE 2.3 Lamotrigine compared with placebo: meta-analysis of randomized trials. *Source: Geddes, Calabrese, and Goodwin (2009).*

could reflect the commonly observed phenomenon of baseline inflation of clinical scores, which would be more likely to affect patients in the less severely ill group as clinicians attempt, probably unconsciously, to make the patients ill enough to participate in the trials.

Finally, one of the main threats to the validity of a systematic review and meta-analysis is publication bias. Although this is recognized early on as the file draw problem by Glass *et al.* when they were first developing meta-analysis, the importance of publication bias has been increasingly recognized and there is substantial concern about the bias estimate of efficacy and safety that it leads to. Evidently, from a marketing point of view, there is less incentive to publish negative or potentially harmful results of an agent and quite often, these studies simply are not published. Although it is possible to infer the presence of publication bias, by methods such as funnel plots, it is now widely considered essential for there to be prospective registration of clinical trials so that all are available to be put in to meta-analysis.

MULTIPLE TREATMENTS META-ANALYSIS

Individual trials can provide reliable estimates of the relative efficacy of an agent versus placebo or against another drug. However, when there is a multiplicity of agents available for the treatment of particular clinical problems such as mania, in the absence of direct comparative evidence, it is very difficult for conclusions to be made about the relative efficacy of treatments. Randomized trials comparing multiple treatment options are rarely feasible. Since the mid-2000s, a new approach to dealing with this has been developed where it is recognized that, if there is a common comparator, unbiased indirect comparisons between interventions across trials can be made (Glenny et al., 2005). A simple approach of indirect comparison can be provided by meta-regression, as performed in the meta-analysis of second-generation antipsychotics in schizophrenia (Geddes et al., 2000). The methods have now evolved into network meta-analysis (or multiple treatments meta-analysis (MTM) or mixed-treatment comparison) in which the direct comparisons of agents within randomized trials are combined with indirect evidence between trials to produce matrices of comparative effectiveness (Cipriani et al., 2013b). These approaches combine direct and indirect evidence. A good example of this is Cipriani et al. who repeated their influential MTM of antidepressant agents (Cipriani et al., 2009) by investigating the relative efficacy of treatments for manic episodes for all registered agents that had antimanic efficacy (Cipriani et al., 2011). This analysis included 68 randomized controlled trials (16,073 participants) published from 1 January 1980 through 25 November 2010, which compared any of aripiprazole, asenapine, carbamazepine, valproate, gabapentin, haloperidol, lamotrigine, lithium, olanzapine, quetiapine, risperidone, topiramate, and ziprasidone at an established therapeutic dose for the treatment of acute mania in adults. The network of comparisons is shown in Figure 2.4.

In Figure 2.4, a line between individual drugs indicates the presence of at least one direct comparison and the width of the trial reflects the number of studies. Therefore, for example, there are relatively large amounts of data on individual drugs versus placebo but very little between active agents. Nonetheless, there are some (e.g., between other drugs and lithium and olanzapine). The olanzapine–placebo comparison and aripiprazole–placebo comparison allow an indirect comparison to be made between olanzapine and aripiprazole (a loop of evidence). The full network is built up from multiple loops and direct evidence is combined with indirect evidence. Network meta-analysis preserve much of the protection from bias derived from randomization because it combines the unbiased between-treatment estimates from individual randomized trials. Nonetheless, it needs to be used cautiously because it crucially depends on the assumption that there are no important differences between the trials making different comparisons, other than the specific treatments being compared. This assumption can be tested by investigating

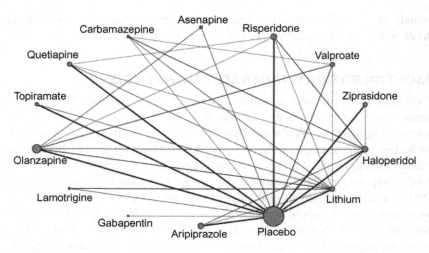

FIGURE 2.4 Comparative efficacy and acceptability of antimanic drugs in acute mania: a multiple-treatments meta-analysis. *Source: Cipriani et al. (2011).*

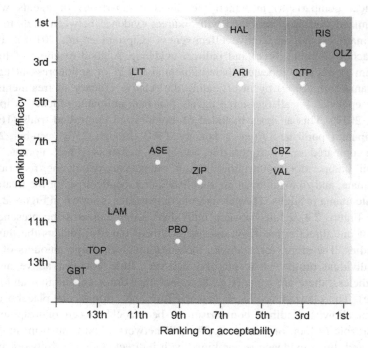

FIGURE 2.5 Ranking of antimanic drugs according to efficacy and acceptability. Red color represents worst treatment and green represents best treatment in a qualitative approach. ARI: aripiprazole; ASE: asenapine; CBZ: carbamazepine; GBT: gabapentin; HAL: haloperidol; LAM: lamotrigine; LIT: lithium; OLZ: olanzapine; PBO: placebo; QTP: quetiapine; RIS: risperidone; TOP: topiramate; VAL: valproate; ZIP: ziprasidone.

the consistency of the results between indirect and direct comparisons and between sets of loops. Just as standard meta-analysis may still serve a useful purpose in demonstrating heterogeneity in the treatment effect between trials even when a pooled mean cannot be calculated, so network meta-analyses can usefully identify possible sources of inconsistency that may include bias and take steps to eradicate it. The results from network analyses can be complex and may best be appreciated visually. Figure 2.5 plots antimanic drugs according to their efficacy and acceptability.

In fact, there are fairly substantial, and clinically relevant, differences between drugs and it can be seen that risperidone and olanzapine have the optimal profiles of available compounds, at least in the short term. Longer-term use will of course depend on estimates of longer-term acceptability and efficacy, which are not provided by this analysis.

CONCLUSIONS

Systematic reviews provide an explicit and reproducible method of synthesizing data and meta-analysis is a powerful method of pooling data between studies when appropriate and identifying and explaining variation between individual studies. Compared with traditional forms of review, systematic reviews are less likely to be subject to bias or to accept apparent advances prematurely. As with most areas of medicine, the clinical management of bipolar disorder has been clarified by the use of systematic reviews.

REFERENCES

Antman, E. M., Lau, J., Kupelnick, B., et al. (1992). A comparison of results of meta-analyses of randomized control trials and recommendations of clinical experts. Treatments for myocardial infarction. *JAMA, 268*(2), 240–248.

Chalmers, I., & Haynes, B. (1994). Reporting, updating, and correcting systematic reviews of the effects of health care. *BMJ, 309*(6958), 862–865.

Cipriani, A., Barbui, C., Salanti, G., et al. (2011). Comparative efficacy and acceptability of antimanic drugs in acute mania: A multiple-treatments meta-analysis. *Lancet, 378*(9799), 1306–13015.

Cipriani, A., Furukawa, T. A., Salanti, G., et al. (2009). Comparative efficacy and acceptability of 12 new-generation antidepressants: A multiple-treatments meta-analysis. *Lancet, 373*(9665), 746–758.

Cipriani, A., & Geddes, J. R. (2003). Comparison of systematic and narrative reviews: The example of the atypical antipsychotics. *Epidemiologica e Psichiatrica Sociale, 12*, 146–154.

Cipriani, A., Hawton, K., Stockton, S., et al. (2013a). Lithium in the prevention of suicide in mood disorders: Updated systematic review and meta-analysis. *BMJ, 346*, f3646–f3646.

Cipriani, A., Higgins, J. P. T., Geddes, J. R., et al. (2013b). Conceptual and technical challenges in network meta-analysis. *Annals of Internal Medicine, 159*, 130–137.

Cipriani, A., Pretty, H., Hawton, K., et al. (2005). Lithium in the prevention of suicidal behaviour and all-cause mortality in patients with mood disorders: A systematic review of randomised trials. *American Journal of Psychiatry, 162*(10), 1805–1819.

Clarke, M. J., & Stewart, L. A. (1994). Obtaining data from randomised controlled trials: How much do we need for reliable and informative meta-analyses? *BMJ, 309*(6960), 1007–1010.

De Angelis, C., Drazen, J. M., Frizelle, F. A., et al. (2004). Clinical trial registration: A statement from the International Committee of Medical Journal Editors. *Lancet*, *364*(9438), 911–912.

Easterbrook, P. J., Berlin, J. A., Gopalan, R., et al. (1991). Publication bias in clinical research. *Lancet*, *337*(8746), 867–872.

Geddes, J. R., Calabrese, J. R., & Goodwin, G. M. (2009). Lamotrigine for treatment of bipolar depression: An independent meta-analysis and meta-regression of individual patient data from five randomised trials. *British Journal of Psychiatry*, *194*(1), 4–9.

Geddes, J. R., Freemantle, N., Harrison, P. J., et al. (2000). Atypical antipsychotics in the treatment of schizophrenia: Systematic review and meta-regression analysis. *BMJ*, *321*, 1371–1376.

Gilbody, S. M., Song, F., Eastwood, A. J., et al. (2000). The causes, consequences and detection of publication bias in psychiatry. *Acta Psychiatrica Scandinavica*, *102*(4), 241–249.

Glenny, A. M., Altman, D. G., Song, F., et al. (2005). Indirect comparisons of competing interventions. *Health Technology Assessment*, *9*(26), 1–134.

Goodwin, F. K., Fireman, B., Simon, G. E., et al. (2003). Suicide risk in bipolar disorder during treatment with lithium and divalproex. *JAMA*, *290*(11), 1467–1473.

Mulrow, C. D. (1987). The medical review article: State of the science. *Annals of Internal Medicine*, *106*(3), 485–488.

Tondo, L., Baldessarini, R. J., Hennen, J., et al. (1998). Lithium treatment and risk of suicidal behavior in bipolar disorder patients. *Journal of Clinical Psychiatry*, *59*(8), 405–414.

Chapter Three

Effectiveness Trials in Bipolar Disorders

Andrew A. Nierenberg

Massachusetts General Hospital; Harvard Medical School, Boston, MA, USA

CHAPTER OUTLINE

EFFICACY VERSUS EFFECTIVENESS: TWO WORDS WITH THE SAME BUT DIFFERENT MEANINGS

As clinicians who treat patients who have bipolar disorder, we make decisions along with our patients everyday about treatment: which treatment to prescribe? When to start? When to stop? When to change? When to persist? While we like to think that we base our decisions on evidence, the literature usually fails to guide us. Why? The majority of randomized clinical trials are efficacy trials that ask questions not relevant to clinical practice. Efficacy trials ask the question, "Will this intervention change the outcome of interest more than placebo?" This is not the question that we ask as clinicians. Instead, we want to know if a treatment will help relieve the suffering of our patients, which treatment to use, and how long to use it for. In contrast to efficacy trials, effectiveness trials ask the question, "How does this intervention work in the actual clinical practice?" (Basu, 2009; Depp & Lebowitz, 2007). Randomized comparative effectiveness studies focus on clinically relevant comparisons to find out which treatment might be better (or at least non-inferior) and which patients may benefit most

Clinical Trial Design Challenges in Mood Disorders. DOI: http://dx.doi.org/10.1016/B978-0-12-405170-6.00003-8

from one treatment compared with another (or more) (Depp & Lebowitz, 2007). Large simple pragmatic trials for interventions for bipolar disorder have been done since the early 2000s and will likely continue, especially with the establishment of the Patient Centered Outcomes Research Network (www.PCOR net.org; last accessed 17 July 2014) and the Mood Patient Powered Research Network (Mood PPRN). The Mood PPRN is meant to serve as a national resource infrastructure that will blend electronic health record data with patient-reported outcomes for a large cohort of 50,000 patients. While ambitious and virtual at the time of the writing of this chapter, it is likely that the Mood PPRN will at least be a platform for prospective comparative effectiveness studies. This chapter will focus on comparative effectiveness studies that inform the care of patients with bipolar disorder.

GENERAL CONSIDERATIONS

In these days of 'Big Data', psychiatric researchers, specifically pharmacoepidemiologists, harvest observational claims data and hospital electronic health records to find patterns and associations that are parallel to findings in prospective comparative effectiveness studies. The difference is that the observational data are not randomized and can be limited by treatment by indication confounding factors. For example, if clinicians prescribe treatment A to patients who are sicker and treatment B to patients who are less sick, if the outcomes for patients who receive treatment A are worse, without measures of baseline severity, it is unknown if treatment A is inferior to treatment B or if the group that received treatment A was more susceptible to have the outcome of interest. This is called susceptibility bias. Randomization minimizes susceptibility bias but can increase volunteer bias compared with observational studies. Volunteer bias refers to potential differences between people who are and people who are not willing to participate in a study. Similarly, invitation bias refers to who the clinician is willing to refer for participation in a study. One glaring example of invitation bias is the almost universal exclusion of bipolar patients who have serious suicidal risk from randomized trials. As a result, most of our treatments for suicidal bipolar patients lack much of an evidence base.

Another limitation in the evidence base for treatment of bipolar disorder is that bipolar disorder is chronic while most randomized studies are short term. Long-term studies tend to be expensive and difficult to conduct because of drop-outs, especially for populations who have serious psychiatric disorders. Shorter-term studies may give some information about the relative worth of competing treatments, with the assumption that such differences, if detected, will persist. Nevertheless, we still have a need for long-term interventional comparative effectiveness studies.

SYSTEMATIC TREATMENT ENHANCEMENT PROGRAM FOR BIPOLAR DISORDER

The systematic treatment enhancement program for bipolar disorder (STEP-BD) provided a system of measurement-based guideline-informed care along with embedded clinical trials (Sachs *et al.*, 2003). Patients could enter STEP-BD as long as they had a diagnosis of bipolar disorder and were willing to be followed. Clinicians were trained to use guideline-informed care as well as track patients' progress using innovative measures along with sharing those measures with patients. Patients were followed for up to 2 years. Among the most informative papers from STEP-BD were those that examined long-term outcomes and the effectiveness of antidepressants added to mood stabilizers.

As for the long-term outcomes, of those who entered STEP-BD and were symptomatic, about 30% reached full recovery (no more than two symptoms that met Diagnostic and Statistical Manual of Mental Disorders, Fourth Edition (DSM-IV) criteria) and were able to stay well (Perlis *et al.*, 2006). Poor prognostic factors included residual manic symptoms that, surprisingly, increased the risk of depressive relapse. Furthermore, patients who were depressed, had residual manic symptoms, and received an antidepressant had similar outcomes to patients who had residual manic symptoms and did not receive an antidepressant (Goldberg *et al.*, 2007). A subset of patients with bipolar depression were randomized to have an antidepressant (either bupropion or paroxetine) or placebo added to a mood stabilizer. The antidepressants provided no advantage over placebo on any measures (Sachs *et al.*, 2007).

Another embedded randomized study examined the outcomes of intensive psychotherapy (interpersonal therapy, cognitive behavioral therapy, or family-focused therapy) compared with psychoeducation for patients with bipolar depression (Miklowitz *et al.*, 2007). Overall, intensive psychotherapy decreased the time to recovery from a bipolar depressive episode by 110 days compared with psychoeducation. An important moderator of this effect appeared to be anxiety, with the advantage of intensive psychotherapy limited to patients who had comorbid anxiety (Deckersbach *et al.*, 2014).

BIPOLAR AFFECTIVE DISORDER: LITHIUM/ ANTICONVULSANT EVALUATION TRIAL

The Bipolar Affective Disorder: Lithium/Anticonvulsant Evaluation (BALANCE) trial examined the effectiveness of continued combination treatment (lithium plus valproate semisodium) compared with monotherapy with either one for those patients who were first stabilized on the combination (Geddes *et al.*, 2010). After a stabilization period of 4–8 weeks, patients were followed for up to 2 years. The combination was better than valproate alone, especially for manic relapse without a substantial difference between combination therapy and lithium alone. No particular advantage was observed for combination therapy over monotherapy for depressive relapse. The essential message from BALANCE is that valproate monotherapy after combination therapy resulted in relatively poor outcomes, especially for manic relapses. However, it is worth mentioning that the overall outcomes were less than desirable, 54% of the combination group, 59% of the lithium group, and 69% of the valproate group required a new intervention for a subsequent mood episode.

DANISH UNIVERSITY ANTIDEPRESSANT GROUP STUDY 6

The Danish University Antidepressant Group study 6 (DUAG-6) examined the effectiveness of lithium compared with lamotrigine for up to 5 years (Licht *et al.*, 2010). Patients with bipolar disorder in a depressive, manic, or mixed episode were first treated at the discretion of clinicians and then randomized to either lithium or lamotrigine. The investigators allowed additional antipsychotic or antidepressant drugs within the first 6 months after randomization. About two-thirds of both groups received antidepressants and about half received antipsychotics in addition to their study medications. Remarkably, no statistically significant differences were found between groups across a wide spectrum of outcomes. Virtually no patients were able to be maintained on monotherapy with lithium or lamotrigine. Antidepressants were added to 72% of the lithium group and 66% of the lamotrigine group; similarly, antipsychotics were added to 54% of the lithium group and 69% of the lamotrigine group.

LITHIUM MODERATE DOSE USE STUDY

The Lithium Moderate Dose Use Study (LiTMUS) was a comparative effectiveness study of optimized personal treatment (OPT) with and without tolerable doses of lithium (called Li + OPT and OPT, respectively) (Nierenberg *et al.*, 2009). The rationale for the study was based on the hypothesis that even low doses of lithium could provide neuroprotection and could potentially improve the outcome of bipolar disorder. OPT allowed for guideline-informed care to be tailored to patients depending on their history and comorbid conditions. In additional to using a global severity scale, LiTMUS also used a novel outcome measure to assess changes in treatment during the trial called necessary clinical adjustments (NCAs). The rationale for NCAs was that clinicians were instructed to get their patients as well as possible and had leeway to prescribe whatever was necessary. If the outcomes between the groups (with and without lithium) were similar, but one group required fewer adjustments over the 6 months of the study, then that group would have been declared superior. However, overall, no statistically significant advantage was observed for Li + OPT (mean ± standard deviation (SD) blood levels 0.47 ± 0.34 meq/L) on the clinical global scale, NCAs, or proportion with sustained remission (26.5% overall; $P = 0.70$). Both groups had similar outcomes across secondary clinical and functional measures. Fewer patients in the Li + OPT group received second-generation antipsychotics (SGA) compared with the OPT alone group (48.3% with Li + OPT vs. 62.5% with OPT).

BIPOLAR CLINICAL HEALTH OUTCOMES INITIATIVE IN COMPARATIVE EFFECTIVENESS TRIAL

The Bipolar Clinical Health Outcomes Initiative in Comparative Effectiveness (Bipolar CHOICE) (Nierenberg *et al.*, 2014) was funded by the Agency for Health Care Research and Quality (AHRQ) to build on LiTMUS. LiTMUS showed that tolerable but low levels of lithium provided minimal benefit when used in the context of OPT. However, lithium has been widely supplanted by the use of SGAs used as mood stabilizers. Thus, it is unknown how lithium at full doses (with levels above 0.6 meq/L) compares to SGAs and whether or not outcomes are improved with SGAs. To this end, Bipolar CHOICE randomized patients with bipolar disorder who were at least mildly ill and who would be willing to take either lithium or quetiapine. The rational for using quetiapine was that it is the only SGA approved to mania and bipolar depression. Again, building on the experience of LiTMUS, the rules of engagement by clinicians were to: 1. treat patients to remission; 2. for patients randomized to lithium, refrain from prescribing any SGA; and 3. for patients randomized to quetiapine, refrain from prescribing lithium or any other SGA. Other treatments could include guideline-informed optimized treatment to manage symptoms and comorbid conditions. Benefits and harms were measured over 6 months, including changes in the Framingham Cardiovascular Risk Score. At the time this chapter was written, the results on Bipolar CHOICE were unavailable.

CONCLUSIONS

Comparative effectiveness studies of treatments for bipolar disorder inform the real world outcomes of evidence-based interventions. So far, we have learned that the outcomes are less than optimal and that it is difficult to show that any treatment or set of treatments have any particular advantage for patients. The results so far cast doubt on the usefulness of antidepressants and the advantages of psychotherapy for patients who have comorbid anxiety disorders. Valproate does not appear to be as useful as once thought. Lithium may very well continue to have a role in the treatment of bipolar disorder and perhaps lamotrigine may be more useful than indicated in efficacy studies. When the results comparing lithium with quetiapine are available, we anticipate that this too will inform clinical care. Future studies should incorporate biomarkers that may allow for better predications of how to match patients and treatments better.

REFERENCES

Basu, A. (2009). Individualization at the heart of comparative effectiveness research: The time for *i*-CER has come. *Medical Decision Making, 29*, N9–N11.

Deckersbach, T., Peters, A. T., Sylvia, L., et al. (2014). Do comorbid anxiety disorders moderate the effects of psychotherapy for bipolar disorder? Results from STEP-BD. *American Journal of Psychiatry, 171*(2), 178–186.

Depp, C., & Lebowitz, B. D. (2007). Clinical trials: Bridging the gap between efficacy and effectiveness. *International Review of Psychiatry, 19*, 531–539.

Geddes, J. R., Goodwin, G. M., Rendell, J., et al. (2010). Lithium plus valproate combination therapy versus monotherapy for relapse prevention in bipolar I disorder (BALANCE): A randomised open-label trial. *Lancet, 375*, 385–395.

Goldberg, J. F., Perlis, R. H., Ghaemi, S. N., et al. (2007). Adjunctive antidepressant use and symptomatic recovery among bipolar depressed patients with concomitant manic symptoms: Findings from the STEP-BD. *American Journal of Psychiatry, 164*, 1348–1355.

Licht, R. W., Nielsen, J. N., Gram, L. F., et al. (2010). Lamotrigine versus lithium as maintenance treatment in bipolar I disorder: An open, randomized effectiveness study mimicking clinical practice. The 6th trial of the Danish University Antidepressant Group (DUAG-6). *Bipolar Disorders, 12,* 483–493.

Miklowitz, D. J., Otto, M. W., Frank, E., et al. (2007). Psychosocial treatments for bipolar depression – A 1-year randomized trial from the systematic treatment enhancement program. *Archives of General Psychiatry, 64,* 419–427.

Nierenberg, A. A., Sylvia, L. G., Leon, A. C., et al. (2009). Lithium treatment-moderate dose use study (LiTMUS) for bipolar disorder: Rationale and design. *Clinical Trials, 6,* 637–648.

Nierenberg, A. A., Sylvia, L. G., Leon, A. C., et al. (2014). Clinical and Health Outcomes Initiative in Comparative Effectiveness for Bipolar Disorder (Bipolar CHOICE): A pragmatic trial of complex treatment for a complex disorder. *Clinical Trials, 11*(1), 114–127.

Perlis, R. H., Ostacher, M. J., Patel, J. K., et al. (2006). Predictors of recurrence in bipolar disorder: Primary outcomes from the systematic treatment enhancement program for bipolar disorder (STEP-BD). *American Journal of Psychiatry, 163,* 217–224.

Sachs, G. S., Nierenberg, A. A., Calabrese, J. R., et al. (2007). Effectiveness of adjunctive antidepressant treatment for bipolar depression. *New England Journal of Medicine, 356,* 1711–1722.

Sachs, G. S., Thase, M. E., Otto, M. W., et al. (2003). Rationale, design, and methods of the systematic treatment enhancement program for bipolar disorder (STEP-BD). *Biological Psychiatry, 53,* 1028–1042.

Chapter Four

Long-Term Treatment of Mood Disorders: Follow-Up of Acute Treatment Phase Studies Versus Continuation and Maintenance Phase Studies, and Enriched Versus Non-Enriched Designs

Willem A. Nolen[1] and Heinz Grunze[2]
[1]*University of Groningen, Groningen, Netherlands;*
[2]*Newcastle University, Newcastle-upon-Tyne, UK*

CHAPTER OUTLINE

Clinical Trial Design Challenges in Mood Disorders. DOI: http://dx.doi.org/10.1016/B978-0-12-405170-6.00004-X

INTRODUCTION

In most patients, mood disorders have a recurrent character and the aim of their treatment should not only be to treat symptoms of acute episodes but also to prevent further episodes. In the literature on the nomenclature of course, treatment, and outcome in mood disorders (Frank *et al.*, 1991; Tohen *et al.*, 2009), a distinction is made between acute treatment phase, continuation treatment phase, and maintenance treatment phase (further referred to as acute, continuation, and maintenance phase). According to a consensus paper supported by the MacArthur Foundation Research Network on the Psychobiology of Depression, for unipolar depression the purpose of the acute phase is to achieve symptomatic response of the acute episode and subsequently remission, whereas the purpose of the continuation phase is to regain full recovery by preventing a return or worsening of the index episode (relapse prevention) (Frank *et al.*, 1991; Figure 4.1). The purpose of the maintenance phase is to prevent new episodes (recurrence prevention) after the patient has achieved recovery, defined in depression as a period of 8 weeks of sustained remission.

Compared with unipolar depression, bipolar disorder is more complex with not only depressive episodes but also (hypo)manic episodes and mixed episodes (or according to Diagnostic and Statistical Manual of Mental Disorders Fifth Edition (DSM-5) episodes with mixed features). This is also reflected in a more complex nomenclature developed by a task force of the International Society for Bipolar Disorders (ISBD; Tohen *et al.*, 2009), as relapse and recurrence can also occur into the opposite pole (Figure 4.2a and b). During the acute and continuation phases, these are called immediate and early switches (in literature also called treatment emergent affective switch (TEAS) as they are often also attributed to treatment), while during the maintenance phase, late switches can be considered as likely recurrences of the opposite pole. Another issue is that the naturalistic course of manic (and mixed) episodes differs from bipolar depressive episodes. As manic episodes tend to be of shorter duration, the duration of the continuation phase in mania (4 weeks) is also shorter than in bipolar depression (8 weeks), which is similar as in unipolar depression.

REQUIREMENTS FOR LICENSING DRUGS IN MOOD DISORDERS

For the license of drugs that are used for the treatment of unipolar depression (major depressive disorder) registration authorities such as the European Medicines Agency (EMA) require both studies showing that they are efficacious

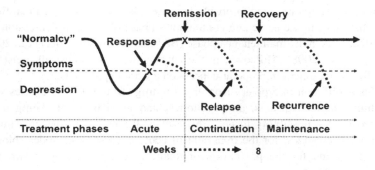

FIGURE 4.1 Nomenclature of treatment phases in unipolar depression. *Source: Frank et al. (1991).*

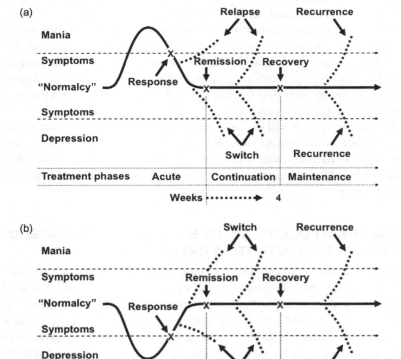

FIGURE 4.2 Nomenclature in bipolar disorder. *Source: Tohen et al. (2009).*

in the treatment of acute episodes and studies showing that their acute effect is maintained in the continuation phase, that is, that they are efficacious in the prevention of relapses (European Medicines Agency, 2013). However, further studies demonstrating their efficacy in the maintenance phase (i.e., the prevention of recurrences) are not required, probably because it is general accepted that those drugs that work in the acute and continuation phase of unipolar depression are also efficacious in the maintenance phase (BALANCE Investigators *et al.*, 2003; Kaymaz *et al.*, 2008). Moreover, in the current situation almost all registered drugs for the treatment of unipolar depression are antidepressants.

This is different in bipolar disorder, with drugs from different classes such as lithium, anticonvulsants, antipsychotics, and antidepressants being used. This creates the possibility to get a license for the treatment of acute manic (and mixed) episodes, for the treatment of acute depressive episodes (bipolar depression), and for the prevention of manic and/or depressive recurrences (maintenance treatment).

Comparable to the license for antidepressants in unipolar depression, the EMA requires that, for the license of drugs for the treatment of an acute manic or bipolar depressive episode, they are efficacious in the acute phase and that their efficacy is maintained during the continuation phase. Efficacy in the continuation phase means that they prevent relapses of the index episode and that they do not increase the likelihood of the occurrence of episodes of the opposite pole (switches) (European Medicines Agency, 2001). For the license of drugs for recurrence prevention (maintenance treatment), studies are required among remitted patients showing that they are efficacious in the prevention of manic and/or depressive recurrences.

In this chapter, we will discuss the major designs that have been used to show efficacy in the continuation phase and maintenance phase of the treatment of mood disorders, with special attention for enriched versus nonenriched designs. The different designs will be illustrated by studies selectively obtained from literature.

LONG-TERM FOLLOW-UP OF RANDOMIZED (PLACEBO-) CONTROLLED ACUTE TREATMENT STUDIES

In this design, the treatment phase is extended beyond the normal duration of the acute phase, which in general is 4–8 weeks in depression and 2–4 weeks in mania (Figure 4.3). A good example is the double-blind, randomized study by McIntyre *et al.* (2005) comparing quetiapine, haloperidol, and placebo for the treatment of acute mania. The study lasted 12 weeks, but the primary end point was change from baseline on the Young Mania Rating Scale (YMRS) at 3 weeks. After these 3 weeks, all participants (i.e., both responders and nonresponders) were followed for a further 9 weeks, while still measuring the effect on mania as well as on depression.

The results showed that both drugs were significantly more effective than placebo at week 3, and that this effect was maintained over the next 9 weeks. Figure 4.4 shows the response rates, defined as a 50% improvement from baseline in the respective rating scale, at every assessment. Overall, patients tended to improve throughout the study, but the vast majority of subjects responded within the first 3 weeks, with significant findings for only haloperidol at

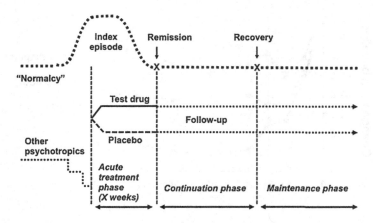

FIGURE 4.3 Usual design of randomized acute treatment phase studies with follow-up.

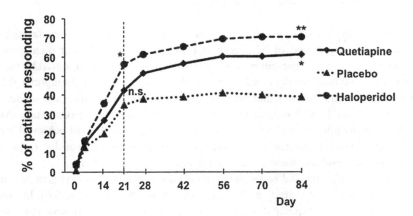

FIGURE 4.4 Response rates in mania study during the acute phase (until week 3) and during follow-up until week 12. *P < 0.05; HAL: haloperidol; n.s.: not significant. *Source: McIntyre et al. (2005).*

week 3 and for both quetiapine and haloperidol at the end of follow-up in comparison with placebo.

Regarding the opposite pole as measured with the Montgomery Åsberg Depression Rating Scale (MADRS), there was no worsening of depressive symptoms with placebo, while with both drugs depression ratings improved significantly for both drugs at week 3, and only for quetiapine at the end of follow-up (Figure 4.5). However, as this trial was conducted in patients with manic only, overall depressive symptom scores were already low at baseline (9.1 quetiapine, 8.3 haloperidol, 9.2 placebo) while, given the overlap of the YMRS and MADRS for some items, this finding could be rather unspecific and should not necessarily be interpreted as a genuine antidepressant effect of the drugs.

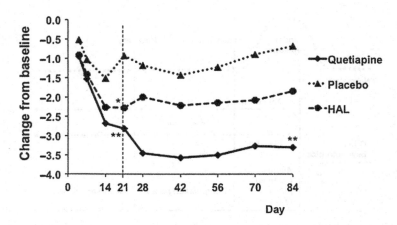

FIGURE 4.5 Change in Montgomery Åsberg Depression Rating Scale (MADRS) ratings in mania study during the acute phase (until week 3) and during follow-up until week 12. * P < 0.05; ** P < 0.01. *Source: McIntyre et al. (2001).*

With this design, one gets an impression of the effects of both drugs throughout the full study period of 12 weeks, but the question of whether quetiapine and haloperidol indeed prevent relapses and switches cannot be answered by this study. First, both responders and nonresponders were followed throughout the study; for the question whether both drugs would prevent relapse and switch, one should have looked only at those who achieved remission from mania. At week 3, remission, defined as a YMRS score of 12 or less, was achieved by 27.7% and 33.6% of the patients treated with quetiapine and haloperidol, respectively, and the results in these patients were not reported separately.

Another study that did report long-term follow-up in responders (but not in remitters) is the LamLit study by Van der Loos *et al.* (2011) (Figure 4.6). In this study, patients with bipolar disorder who had developed a depressive episode during maintenance treatment with lithium were randomized to add-on double-blind treatment with lamotrigine or placebo. Response was defined as a Clinical Global Impression-bipolar version rating (CGI-BP) improvement of depression scale as 2 or less. After 8 weeks (at the end of phase 1), nonresponders received further addition of paroxetine for another 8 weeks (phase 2). Responders during phase 1 or phase 2 were followed up to week 68, or until they developed a relapse or recurrence as indicated by a score of 4 or greater on the CGI-BP severity of depression or mania scale. Patients who had not achieved response during phase 1 or phase 2 dropped out from the study at week 16.

The study allows comparison of two treatments algorithms: lithium plus lamotrigine with or without paroxetine versus lithium plus placebo with or without paroxetine. On the primary outcome measure (change from baseline on the MADRS), the difference between both algorithms (the addition of lamotrigine versus the addition of lithium) was significant at the end of phase 1, but at the end of phase 2 (with the further addition of paroxetine in nonresponders), there was no longer a significant difference.

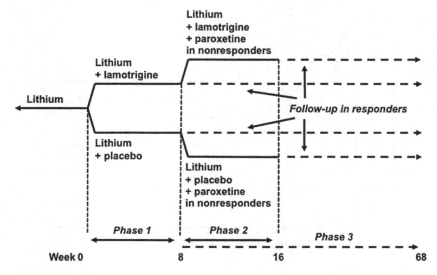

FIGURE 4.6 Design of the LamLit study. *Source: Van der Loos et al. (2011).*

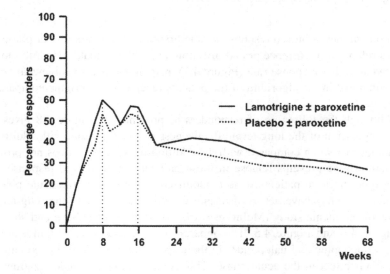

FIGURE 4.7 Responders as percentage of patients who started the study throughout all three phases. *Source: Van der Loos et al. (2011).*

The effects of both treatment algorithms throughout the whole study period of 68 weeks are shown in Figure 4.7 and Figure 4.8. Figure 4.7 shows responders throughout all three phases of the study as a percentage of all patients who entered the study. The figure indicates a somewhat better result of the algorithm with lamotrigine than with placebo.

The follow-up of all patients who achieved response during phase 1 or phase 2 is presented in Figure 4.8. In this analysis, patients were followed from

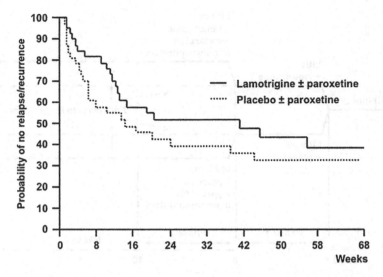

FIGURE 4.8 Probability of maintaining response without relapse/recurrence after having achieved responder status. *Source: Van der Loos et al. (2011).*

the moment they achieved response for the first time during phase 1 or phase 2 until a relapse or recurrence or end of follow-up. It shows that, in addition to a somewhat higher response rate (Figure 4.7), response was also somewhat better maintained in the algorithm of the patients receiving lamotrigine compared with placebo.

Although the follow-up of responders as presented in Figure 4.8 gives a good impression of the long-term effectiveness of the algorithm with addition of lamotrigine when compared with the addition of placebo, it does not prove that lamotrigine prevents relapse in those patients who achieved response to lamotrigine because patients were randomized at the start of the acute phase and not after they have achieved response, which is similar to the long-term follow of the mania study (McIntyre *et al.*, 2005) discussed above and shown in Figure 4.4 and Figure 4.5. The apparent long-term effects of lamotrigine (and of quetiapine and haloperidol in the mania study) may also be explained by its/their effect in the acute phase. This crucial timing of randomization to treatment is different in the studies described in the following chapters.

RANDOMIZED (PLACEBO-)CONTROLLED CONTINUATION PHASE WITHDRAWAL STUDIES

In order to show that the acute effect of a drug is maintained in the continuation phase (i.e., that it is efficacious in the prevention of relapses of the index episode) registration authorities require additional studies in which patients who have achieved remission after acute treatment are randomized to either continuation of the drug or a switch to placebo. Here remission is the entry

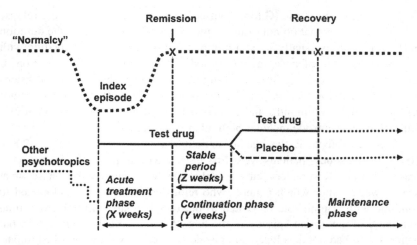

FIGURE 4.9 Usual design of randomized continuation phase withdrawal studies.

criterion for randomization to the respective follow-up treatments and corresponds in these studies with a predefined level and duration of stable euthymia while under treatment. However, operationalization of remission is not uniform and varies widely between studies as far as the symptomatic threshold and the duration are concerned (Grunze *et al.*, 2013). In this so called 'withdrawal design' (or discontinuation design) efficacy during continuation treatment is expressed as the rate of patients relapsing and/or time to relapses or switching to the opposite pole (in bipolar disorder) comparing patients who continued the drug and patients who were allocated to placebo (Figure 4.9).

In the usual design, patients are first treated for an acute (depressive or manic) episode with the study drug usually given open and uncontrolled (so called 'active run-in phase'). Other psychotropic drugs are tapered off, either before or during the acute phase. After patients have achieved predefined criteria for remission or euthymia, open treatment may be continued, usually for some weeks during which the remission status has to be maintained ('stable period' or 'stabilization phase') until randomization and start of follow-up (continuation phase). End point can be (time to) relapse (i.e., return of the index episode) or switch, which can be defined in several ways: fulfilling the full criteria of an episode or a certain score on a severity scale. Another frequently used end point is (time to) 'intervention for an emerging new episode', for example, the perceived need of a clinician to prescribe or change medication in order to prevent deterioration. The latter approach avoids waiting until a full episode has emerged.

The duration of either study phase is hugely variable in the literature. The duration of the stable period (if applied) varies in most studies between 2 and 6 weeks. Together with the criteria for stability (e.g., remission defined as a severity score that is still subsyndromal versus full clinical recovery), this has an impact on the chance to develop a relapse: the longer the stable period, the longer the time to relapse (Gitlin, Abulseoud, & Frye, 2010). For pure relapse prevention studies that do not examine mood episode recurrences, the duration of the follow-up is usually set at a minimum of 6 months, corresponding with the mean duration of a depressive episode. When applying this criterion of mean duration of episode, the follow-up in mania might be shorter, for example, 3 months. However, in practice the follow-up in most continuation studies varies between 6 months and 2 years, which means that the end point of a (emerging) new episode includes both relapse and recurrence.

A good example is the mania continuation study by Keck *et al.* (2006, 2007). In this study, patients were first treated with aripiprazole for an acute manic episode. Responders subsequently entered a stabilization phase of at least 6 weeks, after which patients who remained stable were randomized to continue with aripiprazole or switch to placebo. Primary end point was time to relapse of any mood episode in the first 26 weeks (Keck *et al.*, 2006), but patients who had not developed an episode at week 26 were then asked to participate in a further follow-up of 74 weeks (Keck *et al.*, 2007).

The results clearly showing that all the difference between aripiprazole and placebo was obtained within the first 26 weeks of follow-up (Figure 4.10), indicating efficacy in prevention of relapse, while the difference was maintained during further follow-up. It should however be noted that with this design, efficacy in maintenance treatment, that is, the prevention of recurrences, could not been shown, despite the long-follow-up up to 100 weeks. The drug–placebo difference after week 26 remained unchanged; effective recurrence prevention would be expected to be displayed as a widening of this gap. In contrast, this is also not proof that aripiprazole is ineffective as a recurrence preventive agent. Given the mean length of an untreated manic episode, the natural risk of a manic relapse into the index episode may have leveled out

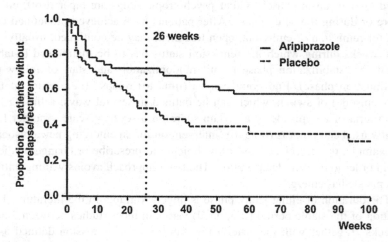

FIGURE 4.10 Results of the mania continuation phase study. *Source: Keck et al. (2006, 2007).*

after 26 weeks, and the remainder of 74 weeks is potentially too short to pick up true prophylactic differences between a drug and placebo in patients who have been stable for more than 6 months. In this respect, it also has to be kept in mind that patients are not on 'no treatment': they receive regular attention and study visits, and the placebo effect has to be taken into account. In this case, a placebo effect may even increase over time, as does the subject's belief to be on effective medication after a prolonged well interval.

RANDOMIZED (PLACEBO-)CONTROLLED MAINTENANCE PHASE WITHDRAWAL STUDIES

As the maintenance phase follows after the continuation phase, that is, starts after the patient has achieved recovery, the stabilization phase of studies investigating the efficacy of drugs in the maintenance phase should extend the continuation phase, which starts after the patient has achieved remission. When we follow the nomenclature as defined by the consensus task forces (Frank *et al.*, 1991; Tohen *et al.*, 2009), this should be in treated patients at least 8 weeks after an index depressive episode and at least 4 weeks after an index manic episode. The rest of the design is similar as in the continuation phase studies (Figure 4.11).

In practice, the distinction between continuation and maintenance studies is clouded, and terms have been used interchangeable, at least in studies in bipolar disorder. Many long-term studies in bipolar disorder include both a continuation and a maintenance element. The outcomes of studies that randomized after a very brief period of remission, for example, the study by Tohen *et al.* (2006), have a marked contribution of early relapses on placebo during, what is still, continuation treatment. The study by Keck *et al.* (2006, 2007), however, randomized patients at a time (6 weeks of stability) where

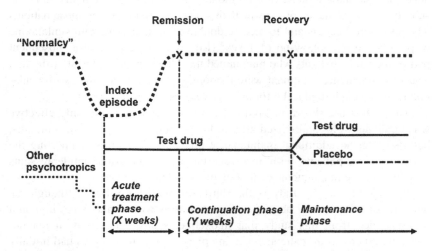

FIGURE 4.11 Usual design of randomized maintenance phase withdrawal studies.

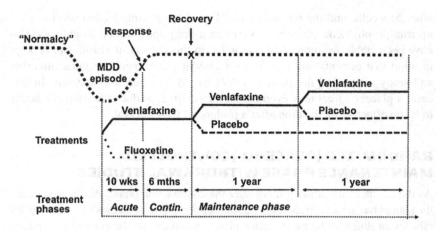

FIGURE 4.12 Design of the venlafaxine maintenance phase studies in unipolar depression. contin: continuation; MDD: major depressive disorder; mths: months; wks: weeks. *Source: Kocsis et al. (2007) and Keller et al. (2007).*

remission from a manic episode has already become recovery, resulting in a low rate of immediate relapses.

An excellent example of a true maintenance phase withdrawal study has been described by Kocsis *et al.* (2007) and Keller *et al.* (2007) (Figure 4.12). In this study, patients with unipolar depression (major depressive disorder) were treated in a double-blind randomized design with venlafaxine or fluoxetine during 10 weeks (acute phase). 'Responders' (defined as a 50% or greater reduction of the 17 items Hamilton Depression Scale (HAM-D-17) at baseline and a total HAM-D-17 score 12 or less) to either drug then received the same drug during a continuation phase of 6 (!) months. The efficacy of venlafaxine in the subsequent maintenance phase was then studied by randomizing those patients who still were 'responders' to receive double-blind treatment with venlafaxine or placebo during follow-up of 1 year (Kocsis *et al.*, 2007). In a subsequent part of the study, patients who maintained their 'responder' status after the first year of maintenance treatment were randomized again to continue with venlafaxine or to switch to placebo for another year (Keller *et al.*, 2007).

The results are shown in Figure 4.13. Venlafaxine was not only effective when patients were randomized after a (long) continuation phase of 6 months, but also after an additional maintenance phase of 12 months, supporting the notion that in patients with recurrent unipolar depression antidepressants remain effective in maintenance treatment for at least 2–3 years.

Remarkable in the study is the third arm with fluoxetine. Although the outcome of this arm did not differ from the arms with venlafaxine, it cannot be concluded from this study that fluoxetine is also efficacious in maintenance treatment, as all patients receiving placebo in both analyses had initially received and responded to venlafaxine and not to fluoxetine.

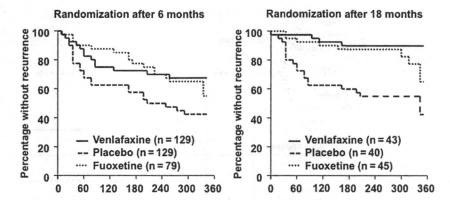

FIGURE 4.13 Time to recurrence during treatment with venlafaxine or placebo in maintenance treatment of unipolar depression 6 months or 18 months after having achieved response. *Source: Kocsis et al. (2007) and Keller et al. (2007).*

ENRICHED VERSUS NONENRICHED DESIGNS

The above-described withdrawal designs for continuation phase and maintenance phase studies are also called enriched designs. At time of randomization, the cohort of patients is enriched with patients who have improved during the preceding open acute phase, that is, who have responded to the drug, and have tolerated the drug. Patients, who did not achieve the respective response (or remission) criteria or have stopped because of adverse effects, do not enter the double-blind continuation or maintenance phase; usually this accounts for 40–60% of all patients who entered the open acute treatment phase. Moreover, the cohort consists of patients who are willing to take medication, both in the acute treatment phase and the subsequent stabilization phase, which results in greater chance that patients will also be compliant with study medication during the subsequent double-blind study period. This results in a greater chance that patients complete the study: thus, increasing the internal validity (or power) of the study to detect a difference between test drug and placebo.

This is not a problem as long as the study has two treatment arms: the test drug and placebo. However, it may become a problem when there is another treatment arm with another drug, for example, the respective standard treatment. An example is the study by Weisler *et al.* (2011) (Figure 4.14).

In this study, 2428 patients were first treated openly with quetiapine for an acute manic, mixed, or depressive episode. Patients who remitted and tolerated the drug then entered a stabilization period of 4 weeks where they had to fulfill remission criteria continuously (YMRS and MADRS score 12 or less). At the end of 4 weeks, this was followed by a maintenance phase in which 1226 patients were randomized to continue with quetiapine or to switch to placebo or, as the third arm, to switch to lithium, which was included in the study as reference intervention.

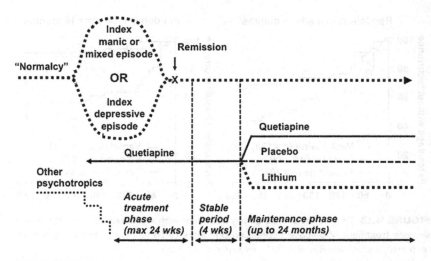

FIGURE 4.14 Design of the study comparing quetiapine and placebo with lithium as standard treatment in the maintenance treatment of bipolar disorder. wks: weeks. *Source: Weisler et al. (2011).*

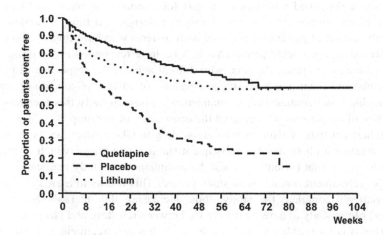

FIGURE 4.15 Result (time to any mood event) of the study comparing quetiapine and placebo with lithium as standard treatment in the maintenance treatment of bipolar disorder. *Source: Weisler et al. (2011).*

The results of the main outcome measure (time to any mood event, Figure 4.15) showed an advantage of both the continuation of quetiapine and switching to lithium over switching to placebo. For quetiapine, this design and outcome is comparable to the withdrawal studies with only one test drug and placebo, as described above. However, the study also 'allows' a comparison of quetiapine versus lithium. Continuation of quetiapine was associated with an advantage over switching to lithium, which, however, should be interpreted with caution,

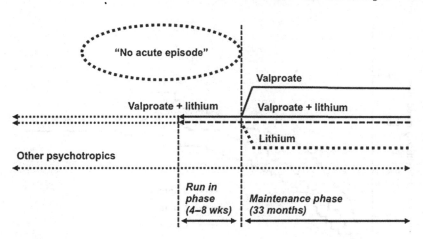

FIGURE 4.16 Design of the study comparing valproate, lithium, and the combination of both drugs in the maintenance treatment of bipolar disorder. wks: weeks. *Source: BALANCE Investigators (2010).*

as the enriched design for quetiapine results in a selection bias in favor of quetiapine, as all patients had both responded to and tolerated quetiapine before randomization. For a fair comparison of quetiapine and lithium, other designs are warranted (see below).

Withdrawal designs with a pre-randomization phase of patients treated with one specific drug followed by an enriched continuation or maintenance phase are not suitable for comparing two active drugs. For a fair comparison, both drugs should be compared in an equal way, either by enriching the study for both drugs, or with a nonenriched design. In addition, studies need to be adequately powered to allow testing for noninferiority, unless the a priori hypothesis is superiority of one drug.

The first option is a design in which patients are first treated with the combination of both drugs, after which patients are randomized to either drug. A good example is the Bipolar Affective Disorder: Lithium/Anticonvulsant Evaluation (BALANCE) effectiveness trial, which compared lithium, valproate, and the combination of both drugs in the maintenance treatment of bipolar disorder (BALANCE Investigators, 2010) (Figure 4.16). This is also almost a true prophylaxis study as patients were euthymic at study entry (run-in phase); however, the protocol did not exclude previous treatment with the investigational drugs, so there is possibly some enrichment as patients in whom lithium or valproate were ineffective/not tolerated in the past were less likely to consent to the study. In this study, patients first received the combination of lithium and valproate in addition to any other ongoing psychotropic medication. Patients adherent to and tolerating both drugs at trial doses during 4–8 weeks were then randomized to open treatment with valproate alone (i.e., withdrawal of lithium), with lithium alone (i.e., withdrawal of valproate), or continuing the combination of valproate and lithium. The design is enriched for both

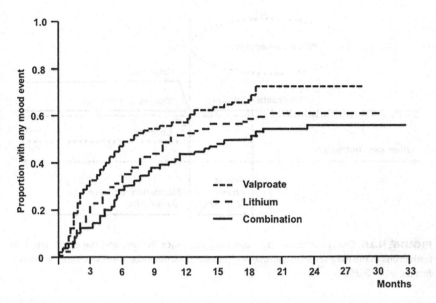

FIGURE 4.17 Results of the study comparing valproate, lithium, and the combination of both drugs in the maintenance treatment of bipolar disorder. *Source: BALANCE Investigators (2010).*

valproate and lithium resulting in a selection of patients willing to take and tolerating both medications.

The results are shown in Figure 4.17. Both the combination and lithium alone were more effective than valproate alone, with no significant difference between the combination and lithium alone. Despite its limitations (no double-blind study, no placebo group, allowing other ongoing psychotropic medication) the importance of this study is that it provides information of the relative effectiveness (value) of two of the most frequently used mood stabilizers, without proving their efficacy (for which a placebo-arm would have been necessary).

The second option is a design in which both drugs are given 'de novo', that is, at randomization patients are not using (or even have never used) any of the drugs. Good examples are two studies comparing lithium and carbamazepine in the maintenance treatment of bipolar disorder, which both found lithium to be more effective than carbamazepine (Greil *et al.*, 1997; Hartong *et al.*, 2003). Both studies included patients who had not been treated prophylactically before (Greil *et al.*, 84%, Hartong *et al.*, 100%) while the last acute episode was also treated with other medication. Lithium or carbamazepine was purely given as a prophylactic drug, while other psychotropic drugs that had been used to treat any previous manic or depressive episode were tapered before start of follow-up.

The rather complicated design of the Hartong *et al.* study is shown in more detail in Figure 4.18. Due to recruitment problems of patients in the original study with randomization only after recovery from the index episode and tapering off other psychotropic medication ('prophylactic randomization';

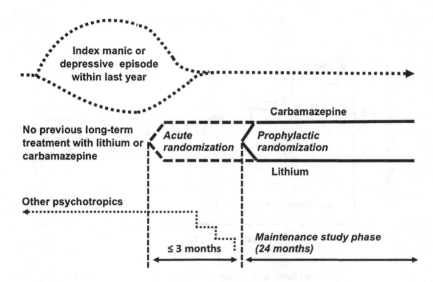

FIGURE 4.18 Design of the partially nonenriched and partially enriched study comparing lithium and carbamazepine in the maintenance treatment of bipolar disorder. *Source: Hartong et al. (2003).*

53 participants), it was decided to also allow randomization during the (end of) the acute phase ('acute randomization'; 41 participants), while the follow-up of these patients started after remission was obtained and other psychotropic drugs were stopped. Actually, this resulted in a partial enriched design as the 'acutely randomized' cohort consisted of patients tolerating the study drug at start of follow-up.

Remarkably, the stratification 'prophylactically randomized' versus 'acutely randomized' appeared to have an impact on the outcome of the study (Figure 4.19a and b). Overall, the patients randomized during the acute phase did respond somewhat better with no significant difference between drugs, than the patients randomized prophylactically with a (nonsignificant) advantage for lithium. As far as we are aware, this is the only study comparing an enriched and nonenriched design within one study. The major limitation is that both parts of the study have insufficient numbers of patients to draw firm conclusions.

CONCLUSION

Various designs have been applied in studying the long-term treatment of mood disorders. It is relevant to differentiate long-term follow-up of acute treatment phase studies from studies investigating efficacy or effectiveness of drugs in the continuation phase and maintenance phase. Nevertheless, the borders between the continuation phase and maintenance phase are arbitrary. Finally, it is relevant to differentiate studies with an enriched design from studies with a nonenriched design, especially when comparing active drugs.

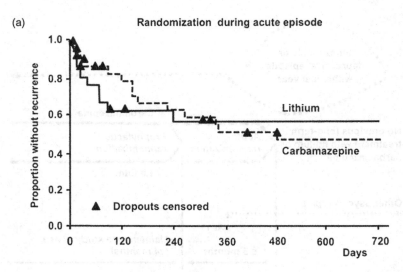

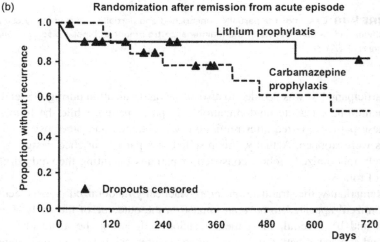

FIGURE 4.19A AND B Results of the partially nonenriched and partially enriched study comparing lithium and carbamazepine in the maintenance treatment of bipolar disorder, stratified according to type of randomization. *Source: Hartong et al. (2003).*

REFERENCES

BALANCE Investigators, Geddes, J. R., Carney, S. M., Davies, C., et al. (2003). Relapse prevention with antidepressant drug treatment in depressive disorders: A systematic review. *Lancet*, *361*(9358), 653–661.

BALANCE Investigators, Geddes, J. R., Goodwin, G. M., Rendell, J., et al. (2010). Lithium plus valproate combination therapy versus monotherapy for relapse prevention in bipolar I disorder (BALANCE): A randomised open-label trial. *Lancet*, *375*(9712), 385–95.

European Medicines Agency. (2001). Note for guidance on clinical investigation of medicinal products for the treatment and prevention of bipolar disorder. <http://www.ema. europa.eu/docs/en_GB/document_library/Scientific_guideline/2009/09/WC500003528. pdf> Last Accessed 19.07.2014.

European Medicines Agency. (2013). Guideline on investigating of medicinal products in the treatment of depression, revision 2. <http://www.ema.europa.eu/docs/en_GB/document_library/Scientific_guideline/2013/05/WC500143770.pdf> Last Accessed 19.07.2014.

Frank, E., Prien, R. F., Jarrett, R. B., et al. (1991). Conceptualization and rationale for consensus definitions of terms in major depressive disorder. Remission, recovery, relapse, and recurrence. *Archives of General Psychiatry, 48*(9), 851–855.

Gitlin, M. J., Abulseoud, O., & Frye, M. A. (2010). Improving the design of maintenance studies for bipolar disorder. *Current Medical Research Opinion, 26*(8), 1835–1842.

Greil, W., Ludwig-Mayerhofer, W., Erazo, N., et al. (1997). Lithium versus carbamazepine in the maintenance treatment of bipolar disorders – a randomised study. *Journal of Affective Disorders, 43*(2), 151–161.

Grunze, H., Vieta, E., Goodwin, G. M., et al. (2013). The World Federation of Societies of Biological Psychiatry (WFSBP) guidelines for the biological treatment of bipolar disorders: Update 2012 on the long-term treatment of bipolar disorder. *World Journal of Biological Psychiatry, 14*, 154–219.

Hartong, E. G., Moleman, P., Hoogduin, C. A., et al. (2003). Prophylactic efficacy of lithium versus carbamazepine in treatment-naive bipolar patients. *Journal of Clinical Psychiatry, 64*(2), 144–151.

Kaymaz, N., van Os, J., Loonen, A. J., et al. (2008). Evidence that patients with single versus recurrent depressive episodes are differentially sensitive to treatment discontinuation: A meta-analysis of placebo-controlled randomized trials. *Journal of Clinical Psychiatry, 69*(9), 1423–1436.

Keck, P. E., Jr., Calabrese, J. R., McIntyre, R. S., et al. (2007). Aripiprazole monotherapy for maintenance therapy in bipolar I disorder: A 100-week, double-blind study versus placebo. *Journal of Clinical Psychiatry, 68*(10), 1480–1491.

Keck, P. E., Jr., Calabrese, J. R., McQuade, R. D., et al. (2006). A randomized, double-blind, placebo-controlled 26-week trial of aripiprazole in recently manic patients with bipolar I disorder. *Journal of Clinical Psychiatry, 67*(4), 626–637.

Keller, M. B., Trivedi, M. H., Thase, M. E., et al. (2007). The Prevention of Recurrent Episodes of Depression with Venlafaxine for Two Years (PREVENT) study: Outcomes from the 2-year and combined maintenance phases. *Journal of Clinical Psychiatry, 68*(8), 1246–1256.

Kocsis, J. H., Thase, M. E., Trivedi, M. H., et al. (2007). Prevention of recurrent episodes of depression with venlafaxine ER in a 1-year maintenance phase from the PREVENT Study. *Journal of Clinical Psychiatry, 68*(7), 1014–1023.

McIntyre, R. S., Brecher, M., Paulsson, B., et al. (2005). Quetiapine or haloperidol as monotherapy for bipolar mania – a 12-week, double-blind, randomised, parallel-group, placebo-controlled trial. *European Neuropsychopharmacology, 15*(5), 573–585.

Tohen, M., Calabrese, J. R., Sachs, G. S., et al. (2006). Randomized, placebo-controlled trial of olanzapine as maintenance therapy in patients with bipolar I disorder responding to acute treatment with olanzapine. *American Journal of Psychiatry, 163*, 247–256.

Tohen, M., Frank, E., Bowden, C. L., et al. (2009). The International Society for Bipolar Disorders (ISBD) Task Force report on the nomenclature of course and outcome in bipolar disorders. *Bipolar Disorders, 11*(5), 453–473.

Van der Loos, M. L., Mulder, P., Hartong, E. G., et al. (2011). Long-term outcome of bipolar depressed patients receiving lamotrigine as add-on to lithium with the possibility of the addition of paroxetine in nonresponders: A randomized, placebo-controlled trial with a novel design. *Bipolar Disorders, 13*(1), 111–117.

Weisler, R. H., Nolen, W. A., Neijber, A., et al. (2011). Continuation of quetiapine versus switching to placebo or lithium for maintenance treatment of bipolar I disorder (Trial 144: A randomized controlled study). *Journal of Clinical Psychiatry, 72*(11), 1452–1464.

Chapter Five

The Role of Noninferiority Designs in Bipolar Disorder Clinical Trials

Eduard Vieta and Núria Cruz

University of Barcelona, Barcelona, Spain

CHAPTER OUTLINE

INTRODUCTION

A randomized controlled trial is the classical tool that is used to establish the differences between two treatments (or between a treatment and a placebo) (Kabisch *et al.*, 2011), with the aim of demonstrating that a certain (usually novel) treatment option is superior to the existing standard. In dealing with diseases for which adequate treatment options are already available, the new drug is developed to ameliorate adverse effects and/or to improve efficacy. In that case, and particularly when superiority is not expected, the aim is to test the hypothesis that the efficacy of the new drug, compared with existing

Clinical Trial Design Challenges in Mood Disorders. DOI: http://dx.doi.org/10.1016/B978-0-12-405170-6.00005-1

reference medications, is essentially similar (equivalence) or only marginally lower at most (noninferiority).

In medicine, most active control trials are currently planned and evaluated on the basis of noninferiority tests (Wellek & Blettner, 2012). From the point of view of statistical theory, there are no compelling reasons for this preference. Rather, it is motivated by the fact that given the same lower margin of equivalence and the same desired power, considerably higher sample sizes are needed to establish noninferiority versus superiority. Moreover, each type of trial requires different procedures for statistical analysis and specific publications reporting requirements summarized in the Consolidated Standards of Reporting Trials (CONSORT) Statement (Piaggio *et al.*, 2006). In psychiatry, superiority designs are preferred because effect sizes are not consistent across trials (Vieta & Cruz, 2012). Another relevant concern, especially in psychiatry, is that placebo-controlled trials have been criticized as being ethically controversial in clinical situations where effective treatment options are available (Baldwin *et al.*, 2003; Carpenter, Schooler, & Kane, 1997; Fritze & Möller, 2001; Laporte & Figueras, 1994). More restrictions to the use of placebo were exposed by regulatory agencies in schizophrenia guideline documents (CPMP/ EWP/559/95; CPMP, 1998) when comparing with those for bipolar disorder (CPMP/EWP/567/98; CPMP, 2001) or depression (CPMP/EWP/ 518/97 Rev.1; CPMP, 2002), owing to potentially irreversible harms as a result of restricting access to effective treatment to patients with schizophrenia. However, the majority of placebo-controlled trials in schizophrenia and most psychiatric conditions show slight, but real benefits, rather than harm, for the patients randomized to placebo (Dunn, Candilis, & Roberts, 2006; Kotzalidis *et al.*, 2008; Tedeschini *et al.*, 2010). In psychiatry, worsening when taking placebo is relatively rare (Vieta & Carne, 2005; Wyatt, Henter, & Bartko, 1999), and no significant increase in mortality has been shown (Isaac & Koch, 2010). On the contrary, the perception that head-to-head trials are more ethical and safe for the patients may be wrong, especially in the case of noninferiority designs, because they expose many more patients to the experimental drug and they might allow the approval of progressively weak or even ineffective drugs into the market. Nevertheless, some academics support the general recommendation that studies with potential new antidepressants or antipsychotics should employ only a comparator-controlled design, whereby new drugs have to be noninferior or superior to existing treatment (Fleischhacker *et al.*, 2003). From a regulatory perspective though, it becomes clear that restricting approval to drugs that prove to be superior to licensed drugs may hinder access of effective agents that may not be more efficacious but actually safer or more tolerable than the available drugs. Allowing noninferiority as proof of efficacy may be too permissive, yielding approval to very weak drugs with questionable benefit–risk ratios.

TRIALS FOR DRUG REGISTRATION VERSUS TRIALS THAT ARE MOST CLINICALLY INFORMATIVE

Why Superiority Designs are Preferred by Regulators in the Field of Bipolar Disorder

Newly developed drugs often do not have better efficacy, in terms of superiority, or the absence of biomarkers/hard variables makes it difficult to prove that they do. This is the reason for the need of placebo, especially in psychopharmacology (Vieta & Cruz, 2008; Walsh *et al.*, 2002; Yildiz *et al.*, 2011a). Thus, no regulatory authority demands proof of superiority over available treatment options as a requirement for licensing in psychiatry. Otherwise, compounds with the only novelty of new mechanisms of action but no increased efficacy could not be submitted for marketing authorization losing the opportunity to find more specific approaches for patient subgroups (Möller & Broich, 2010). Superiority studies comparing two active drugs, though, may be very relevant as postmarketing approval information, but given their risks, cost, and limited extra value from an industry perspective, they are rarely conducted by private sponsors. Examples of superiority comparative trials are the CATIE (Clinical Antipsychotic Trials for Intervention Effectiveness) study for schizophrenia (Lieberman *et al.*, 2005), which was sponsored by the US National Institute of Mental Health, and, in bipolar disorder, the aripiprazole–haloperidol trial (Vieta *et al.*, 2005). A further issue with head-to-head studies, which may be especially relevant when such studies are industry-sponsored, is the choice of the primary outcome, target dose, titration, and concomitant medication. Even geographical and cultural factors may play a role in differential response to active drugs (Vieta *et al.*, 2011). While the trial design of regulatory placebo-controlled trials is quite well established, in the absence of placebo there is the potential risk that known or unknown shortcomings in selecting the dose for the active comparator, for example, might bias the results. This has happened quite often with industry-sponsored postmarketing studies that were used as a strategy to show advantages over competitors (Heres *et al.*, 2006; Vieta, 2007).

The Need of Clinically Informative Designs: Alternatives to Superiority Observational and Exploratory Trials

With the only accomplishment of the 50% response criterion, no information is provided about what treatment options may be required in order to achieve a more sustained response or the ideal goal of remission. This is increasingly an important goal because considerable data indicate that subsyndromal symptomatology of any polarity is a poor prognosis indicator and predicts newer recurrences in the near future (Judd *et al.*, 2002; Perlis *et al.*, 2006). Moreover, relapse prevention trials generally use time to any mood episode as primary outcome, which does not inform about long-term outcome beyond the mood event.

Furthermore, while there is wide recognition that the use of multiple drugs in combination is the rule for bipolar outpatients, the drugs are almost invariably initially studied for regulatory approval as monotherapy, and, more recently but still rarely, dual drug combination. Clinical trial designs have not yet included those needed to help elucidate the best sequences of drugs to be tried and the combinations most likely to be effective (Post & Luckenbaugh, 2003; Sachs, 2001).

In additional, real-world complex patients with anxiety and substance abuse comorbidities are typically excluded from clinical trials, independently of the design. Most trials are often extremely short term, when assessing efficacy in acute phases, ranging from 3 to 8 weeks, which does not allow sufficient time to assess the true magnitude of initial drug effect or requirement for more complex augmentation strategies. In summary, clinicians are more interested in sustained rather than transient responses.

NONINFERIORITY DESIGNS

The importance of equivalence and noninferiority studies for clinical research in medicine has increased steadily since the 1990s, as can be seen from the number of PubMed hits for the search terms 'bioequivalence', '(non)inferiority study (trial)', and 'equivalence study (trial)' over the years 1991–2011 (Figure 5.1) (Wellek & Blettner, 2012). Another indicator for this development

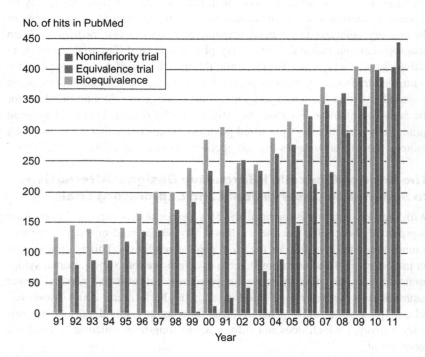

FIGURE 5.1 Frequency of equivalence trials: results of a literature search. *Source: Adapted with permission from Wellek and Blettner (2012).*

is the proportion of drugs approved for the market on the basis of equivalence trials. According to an extrapolation from data in drug reports published by the US Food and Drug Administration (FDA), this proportion was as high as 78% in 2008 (Figure 5.1; Wellek & Blettner, 2012). However, regulatory agencies do not advise noninferiority designs in psychiatry, and there are few pivotal trials that have used this strategy. One example in psychopharmacology is the noninferiority extension trial comparing asenapine with olanzapine in mania (Cruz & Vieta, 2011; McIntyre *et al.*, 2009).

Because the intent of the trial is one-sided (i.e., to show that the new drug is not materially worse than the control), they are now called noninferiority trials (US Department of Health and Human Services, 2010). In fact, that can be considered a misnomer because guaranteeing that the test drug is not any (even a little) less effective than the control can only be demonstrated by showing that the test drug is superior. What noninferiority trials seek to show is that any difference between the two treatments is small enough to allow a conclusion that the new drug has at least some effect or, in many cases, an effect that is not too much smaller than the active control. By defect, this procedure assumes that the chosen reference drug really is superior to placebo at an effective dose. However, this is not self-evident. For example, half of placebo-controlled studies of an antidepressant generally accepted to be efficacious will fail to show superiority over placebo (US Department of Health and Human Services, 2010). This is not exclusive of antidepressant drugs: failed trials have been reported in schizophrenia (Citrome, 2009) and in mania (El Mallakh *et al.*, 2010; Yildiz *et al.*, 2011b) with antipsychotics that appeared to work well in several other studies. Thus, even if the study drug appears to be effective in the equivalence/noninferiority test, it cannot be ruled out that the study has failed (i.e., that in this study both drugs were (similarly) ineffective, e.g., due to lack of assay sensitivity of the trial) (Leon, 2011). Researchers who advocate the use of noninferiority designs as opposed to placebo-controlled trials in certain conditions, such as schizophrenia (Fleischhacker *et al.*, 2003), argue that the mean effect of placebo can be calculated from meta-analyses, giving solid grounds for the implementation of a reliable noninferiority margin; however, there are also indications of progressive increase of placebo response over time not only in depression (Walsh *et al.*, 2002), but also in mania (Sysko & Walsh, 2007) and schizophrenia (Kemp *et al.*, 2010), and it has been reported that the placebo response may vary depending on the specific study design and number of comparator arms (Rutherford, Sneed, & Roose, 2009; Sinyor *et al.*, 2010) making the assumption that placebo response can be extrapolated from one set of trials to another even more questionable. Finally, there is still the risk that a poorly performed trial might look like a positive noninferiority study, due to uncertain assay sensitivity.

For all the reasons discussed above, noninferiority trials appear to be far from ideal for regulatory purposes, and in our opinion, superiority trials (in most cases, placebo-controlled studies) are still necessary; they are not ideal either, but still better, from both ethical and methodologic grounds, than noninferiority.

Table 5.1 Advantages, Disadvantages, Alternatives, and Practical Use of Noninferiority Trials in Bipolar Disorder

Advantages

Comparative effectiveness data

Large safety data

Higher generalizability vs. placebo-controlled trial

Can provide further information on assay sensitivity when combined with placebo superiority designs (three or more arm studies)

May help in guiding cost-effectiveness decisions (comparative efficiency)

Disadvantages

Relies on evidence from other studies for the comparator (superiority trials)

Uncertain assay sensitivity

Assumes that historical differences between active comparator and placebo are constant

Noninferiority margin may be clinically questionable

Large sample exposure to experimental (potentially ineffective or unsafe) drug

May allow registration of very weak or even ineffective drugs

May indirectly promote approval of progressively weaker drugs (if every new drug is compared with the weakest available: this is termed 'Biocreep')

May indirectly promote poor-quality studies (which are more likely to show no differences between treatments)

More lengthy and expensive than placebo-controlled studies

Alternatives

Superiority vs. placebo trials

Superiority vs. comparator trials

Add-on superiority trials

Fixed-dose (superiority vs. low dose) trials

Adaptive mixed designs (adaptive three-arm trial combining superiority and noninferiority)

Practical use

In combination with a placebo-superiority design in three-arm studies

As a supplement to regulatory superiority trials (for approved drugs and indications)

For cost-effectiveness studies

Source: Adapted with permission from Vieta and Cruz (2012).

However, noninferiority studies do have a place because they may provide potentially useful information on comparative effectiveness, safety data, and cost-effectiveness. A combined design, which is feasible and informative, is that of a three-arm study with a placebo arm, an experimental drug arm, and a comparator arm. The trial can be powered for superiority over placebo and for noninferiority versus the active compound.

CONCLUSIONS

Data from noninferiority studies has an independent entity. They need to be assessed for statistical significance no less than data that are generated to show that two treatments have different effects. A negative result in a traditional two-sided test does not suffice for statistically proving equivalence. In addition, considering all the methodologic and ethical concerns explained above, placebo-controlled studies of new psychopharmacologic agents are still justified and necessary, both ethically and scientifically for all psychiatric conditions, and particularly for bipolar disorder. Superiority designs are the only designs that exert compelling evidence of efficacy and assay sensitivity, and if placebo has to be avoided, superiority head-to-head studies can be conducted, using either a placebo or a 'weak' comparator. There is no reason, though, to avoid noninferiority for secondary measures, the only caveat being, in most cases, statistical power issues. Finally, noninferiority designs may not be scientifically powerful enough to be used for regulatory purposes, although they may yield clinically relevant information on comparative safety and cost-effectiveness. Their applications should address clinical information about the comparable effectiveness versus an active control currently available. An overview of noninferiority trials is given in Table 5.1.

REFERENCES

Baldwin, D., Broich, K., Fritze, J., et al. (2003). Placebo-controlled studies in depression: Necessary, ethical and feasible. *European Archives of Psychiatry and Clinical Neuroscience, 253*, 22–28.

Carpenter, W. T., Jr., Schooler, N. R., & Kane, J. M. (1997). The rationale and ethics of medication-free research in schizophrenia. *Archives of General Psychiatry, 54*, 401–407.

Citrome, L. (2009). Asenapine for schizophrenia and bipolar disorder: A review of the efficacy and safety profile for this newly approved sublingually absorbed second-generation antipsychotic. *International Journal of Clinical Practice, 63*, 1762–1784.

CPMP. (1998). *Notes for guidance on the clinical investigation of medicinal products in the treatment of schizophrenia.* <http://www.ema.europa.eu/docs/en_GB/document_library/Scientific_guideline/2009/09/WC500003541.pdf/> Accessed 25.07.14.

CPMP. (2001). *Notes for guidance on the clinical investigation of medicinal products in the treatment of bipolar disorder.* <http://www.ema.europa.eu/docs/en_GB/document_library/Scientific_guideline/2009/09/WC500003528.pdf/> Accessed 25.07.14.

CPMP. (2002). *Notes for guidance on the clinical investigation of medicinal products in the treatment of depression.* <http://www.ema.europa.eu/docs/en_GB/document_library/Scientific_guideline/2009/09/WC500003526.pdf/> Accessed 25.07.14.

Cruz, N., & Vieta, E. (2011). Asenapine: A new focus on the treatment of mania. *Revista de Psiquiatría y Salud Mental, 4*, 101–108.

Dunn, L. B., Candilis, P. J., & Roberts, L. W. (2006). Emerging empirical evidence on the ethics of schizophrenia research. *Schizophrenia Bulletin, 32*, 47–68.

El Mallakh, R. S., Vieta, E., Rollin, L., et al. (2010). A comparison of two fixed doses of aripiprazole with placebo in acutely relapsed, hospitalized patients with bipolar disorder I (manic or mixed) in subpopulations (CN138-007). *European Neuropsychopharmacology, 20*, 776–783.

Fleischhacker, W. W., Czobor, P., Hummer, M., et al. (2003). Placebo or active control trials of antipsychotic drugs? *Archives of General Psychiatry, 60*, 458–464.

Fritze, J., & Möller, H. J. (2001). Design of clinical trials of antidepressants: Should a placebo control arm be included? *CNS Drugs, 15*, 755–764.

Heres, S., Davis, J., Maino, K., et al. (2006). Why olanzapine beats risperidone, risperidone beats quetiapine, and quetiapine beats olanzapine: An exploratory analysis of head-to-head comparison studies of second-generation antipsychotics. *American Journal of Psychiatry, 163*, 185–194.

Isaac, M., & Koch, A. (2010). The risk of death among adult participants in trials of antipsychotic drugs in schizophrenia. *European Neuropsychopharmacology, 20*, 139–145.

Judd, L. L., Akiskal, H. S., Schettler, P. J., et al. (2002). The long-term natural history of the weekly symptomatic status of bipolar I disorder. *Archives of General Psychiatry, 59*, 530–537.

Kabisch, M., Ruckes, C., Seibert-Grafe, M., et al. (2011). Randomized controlled trial: Part 17 of a series on evaluation of scientific publications. *Deutsches Ärzteblatt International, 108*, 663–668.

Kemp, A. S., Schooler, N. R., Kalali, A. H., et al. (2010). What is causing the reduced drug-placebo difference in recent schizophrenia clinical trials and what can be done about it? *Schizophrenia Bulletin, 36*, 504–509.

Kotzalidis, G., Pacchiarotti, I., Manfredi, G., et al. (2008). Ethical questions in human clinical psychopharmacology: Should the focus be on placebo administration? *Journal of Psychopharmacology, 22*, 590–597.

Laporte, J. R., & Figueras, A. (1994). Placebo effects in psychiatry. *Lancet, 344*, 1206–1209.

Leon, A. (2011). Comparative effectiveness clinical trials in psychiatry: Superiority, noninferiority, and the role of active comparators. *Journal of Clinical Psychiatry, 72*, 1344–1349.

Lieberman, J. A., Stroup, S. T., McEvoy, J. P., et al. (2005). Effectiveness of antipsychotic drugs in patients with chronic schizophrenia. *New England Journal of Medicine, 353*, 1209–1223.

McIntyre, R. S., Cohen, M., Zhao, J., et al. (2009). Asenapine versus olanzapine in acute mania: A double-blind extension study. *Bipolar Disorders, 11*, 815–826.

Möller, H. J., & Broich, K. (2010). Principle standards and problems regarding proof of efficacy in clinical psychopharmacology. *European Archives of Psychiatry and Clinical Neuroscience, 260*, 3–16.

Perlis, R. H., Ostacher, M. J., Patel, J. K., et al. (2006). Predictors of recurrence in bipolar disorder: Primary outcomes from the Systematic Treatment Enhancement Program for Bipolar Disorder (STEP-BD). *American Journal of Psychiatry, 179*, 286–287.

Piaggio, G., Elbourne, D. R., Altman, D. G., et al. (2006). Reporting of non-inferiority and equivalence randomized trials: An extension of the CONSORT statement. *JAMA, 295*, 1152–1160.

Post, R. M., & Luckenbaugh, D. A. (2003). Unique design issues in clinical trials of patients with bipolar affective disorder. *Journal of Psychiatric Research, 37*, 61–73.

Rutherford, B. R., Sneed, J. R., & Roose, S. P. (2009). Does study design influence outcome? The effects of placebo control and treatment duration in antidepressant trials. *Psychotherapy and Psychosomatics, 78*, 172–181.

Sachs, G. S. (2001). Design and promise of NIMH multicenter effectiveness trials: A STEP forward. *Bipolar Disorders, 3*(Suppl. 1), 16–17.

Sinyor, M., Levitt, A. J., Cheung, A. H., et al. (2010). Does inclusion of a placebo arm influence response to active antidepressant treatment in randomized controlled trials? Results from pooled and meta-analyses. *Journal of Clinical Psychiatry, 71*, 270–279.

Sysko, R., & Walsh, B. T. (2007). A systematic review of placebo response in studies of bipolar mania. *Journal of Clinical Psychiatry, 68*, 1213–1217.

Tedeschini, E., Fava, M., Goodness, T. M., et al. (2010). Relationship between probability of receiving placebo and probability of prematurely discontinuing treatment in double-blind, randomized clinical trials for MDD: A meta-analysis. *European Neuropsychopharmacology, 20*, 527–562.

US Department of Health and Human Services. (2010). *Food and Drug Administration; Center for Drug Evaluation and Research (CDER); Center for Biologics Evaluation and Research (CBER). Guidance for industry non-inferiority trials.* <http://www.fda. gov/downloads/drugs/guidancecomplianceregulatoryinformation/guidances/ucm202140. pdf/> Accessed 23.07.14.

Vieta, E. (2007). Psychiatry: From interest in conflicts to conflicts of interest. *World Psychiatry, 6,* 27–29.

Vieta, E., Bourin, M., Sanchez, R., et al. (2005). Effectiveness of aripiprazole v. haloperidol in acute bipolar mania: Double-blind, randomised, comparative 12-week trial. *British Journal of Psychiatry, 187,* 235–242.

Vieta, E., & Carne, X. (2005). The use of placebo in clinical trials on bipolar disorder: A new approach for an old debate. *Psychotherapy and Psychosomatics, 74,* 10–16.

Vieta, E., & Cruz, N. (2008). Increasing rates of placebo response over time in mania studies. *Journal of Clinical Psychiatry, 69,* 681–682.

Vieta, E., & Cruz, N. (2012). Head to head comparisons as an alternative to placebo-controlled trials. *European Neuropsychopharmacology, 22,* 800–803.

Vieta, E., Pappadopulos, E., Mandel, F. S., et al. (2011). Impact of geographical and cultural factors on clinical trials in acute mania: Lessons from a ziprasidone and haloperidol placebo-controlled study. *International Journal of Neuropsychopharmacology, 14,* 1017–1027.

Walsh, B. T., Seidman, S. N., Sysko, R., et al. (2002). Placebo response in studies of major depression: Variable, substantial, and growing. *JAMA, 287,* 1840–1847.

Wellek, S., & Blettner, M. (2012). Establishing equivalence or non-inferiority in clinical trials. *Deutsches Ärzteblatt International, 109,* 674–679.

Wyatt, R. J., Henter, I. D., & Bartko, J. J. (1999). The long-term effects of placebo in patients with chronic schizophrenia. *Biological Psychiatry, 46,* 1092–1105.

Yildiz, A., Vieta, E., Leucht, S., et al. (2011b). Efficacy of antimanic treatments: Meta-analysis of randomized, controlled trials. *Neuropsychopharmacology, 36,* 375–389.

Yildiz, A., Vieta, E., Tohen, M., et al. (2011a). Factors modifying drug and placebo responses in randomized trials for bipolar mania. *International Journal of Neuropsychopharmacology, 14,* 863–875.

Chapter Six

The Use of Mixed Methods in Drug Discovery: Integrating Qualitative Methods into Clinical Trials

Michael Berk,[1,2,3,4] Renée Otmar,[1] Olivia Dean,[1,2] Lesley Berk[1,2] and Erin Michalak[5]

[1]*Deakin University, School of Medicine, Geelong, VIC, Australia;* [2]*The University of Melbourne, Parkville, VIC, Australia;* [3]*Florey Institute for Neuroscience and Mental Health, Parkville, VIC, Australia;* [4]*Centre for Youth Mental Health, Parkville, VIC, Australia;* [5]*University of British Columbia, Vancouver, BC, Canada*

CHAPTER OUTLINE

Clinical Trial Design Challenges in Mood Disorders. DOI: http://dx.doi.org/10.1016/B978-0-12-405170-6.00006-3

INTRODUCTION

The primary scientific process used in the evaluation of a putative psychotropic agent involves the generation of the hypothesis, formulation of a strategy for the evaluation of that hypothesis, and formal testing of the hypothesis in the context of a clinical trial. For the hypothesis of interest to be tested, usually a clinical syndrome's response to an agent of interest, rating instruments that are specific to that hypothesis are selected. There is no argument as to the fundamental role of this pathway of investigation. However, this approach, despite being considered the most rigorous for use in detecting the effect of an agent on the disorder of interest, delivers very poor results when used to detect unexpected, novel, or latent associations in datasets.

In this chapter, we contend that clinical trial methodologies can be usefully augmented with research methods that are hypothesis-generating, able to detect covert, or latent, factors that might emerge in the conduct of a clinical trial, and provide indepth understanding of phenomena, including behaviors. Such mixed-method (or multi-method) approaches take a wide view of science's systematic and empirical search for knowledge by combining complementary methods from quantitative and qualitative research methodologies. To use an optical analogy, it is possible to gain a far broader perspective using a wide-angle lens than a microscope, but using both offers the combined values of scope and detail, and thus deeper understanding of the phenomena under investigation.

We begin with a rationale for mixed-method approaches in the design of clinical trials. Along with a definition of qualitative research, we describe a sample of qualitative methodologic frameworks and methods that may serve as exemplars of potential utility in the context of clinical trials. We conclude the chapter with an example of a study in which this method was successfully applied.

A RATIONALE FOR MIXED-METHOD APPROACHES TO CLINICAL TRIAL DESIGN

One of the great limitations of psychiatric research is the absence of a coherent and validated pathophysiology for any of the major neuropsychiatric disorders. In disorders in which there is a clear molecular target; that is, a true biomarker of the disorder of interest exists, there is far greater validity in the selection of pharmacologic probes than in disorders in which a biomarker is not extant. The absence of biomarker targets in neuropsychiatry makes the process of drug discovery far more random. There is no good way to predict, for example, that an agent working on glutamate, substance P, corticotrophin-releasing hormone, or any other biomarker of interest could be translated into a pharmacotherapeutic agent that might be operative in a particular psychiatric disorder. Indeed, it could be argued that singular reliance on the traditional clinical trial method greatly restricts the ability to detect hidden associations, patterns, and properties in clinical trial datasets.

The above is all the more salient in the context of the history of drug discovery in psychiatry. Almost all psychotropics considered useful today in clinical therapy have been discovered serendipitously. A case in point is lithium, the clinical utility of which was not realized until more than a century after its first discovery in Sweden in 1817. Tricyclics and antipsychotics were first synthesized as antihistamines in the early decades of the 20th century, in similarly fortuitous circumstances. Likewise, the monoamine oxidase inhibitors were first synthesized as antibiotics from the 1940s onward and into the 1990s.

Furthermore, it could be argued that much of our current understanding of neuropathology is based on reverse engineering of the biologic effects of agents discovered serendipitously. As a consequence, even this knowledge is limited by boundary issues: it remains unclear to what extent knowledge of an agent's biologic effects provides a true reflection of underlying disorder, or instead whether such effects are merely part of a subset of the biologic components upon which the agent of interest has an action. In the field of clinical trials, it is clear that we need to leverage the potential of such serendipity, thereby maximizing capacity to discover useful, latent, and unexpected properties of agents whenever they are studied.

It has been observed that "drug discovery is at a near stand-still for treating psychiatric disorders such as schizophrenia, bipolar disorder, depression and common forms of autism" (Hyman, 2012, p. 155). In light of this, we propose that the use of hypothesis-generating techniques may assist in detecting associations indicating potential efficacy of agents in unexpected symptom patterns. We argue that far greater emphasis needs to be placed on the generation of hypotheses in the context of clinical trials than has been the case to date. The integration of qualitative research into clinical trial design has the potential to assist with this goal.

Qualitative research, by its very nature, can be used to observe patterns and phenomena in situ as well as in extant datasets, and, unlike quantitative methods, is often utilized in order to generate hypotheses rather than test them.

QUALITATIVE RESEARCH DEFINED

Qualitative research studies typically seek to answer questions about the 'what', 'how', and 'why' of phenomena. This is in contrast to the questions of 'how many' or 'how much' that are sought to be answered by quantitative research, including epidemiologic studies and clinical trials. A common distinguishing feature of qualitative research is that studies often aim to explore and understand, rather than measure phenomena and behaviors (Green & Thorogood, 2004).

In the context of medical and health research, qualitative studies may seek to investigate phenomena from the perspective of stakeholders, such as individuals or communities affected by health, illness, or health services, or the professionals who provide those health services. The qualitative strand of a large health research study may be exploratory (pilot), as a precursor to other research designs, or may follow quantitative research to provide depth to findings or to explore the meaning of those findings (Green & Thorogood, 2004).

Given its roots in early American sociology and anthropology (Liamputtong, 2009), qualitative research is underpinned by theory (Green & Thorogood, 2004). Theoretical perspectives on the role of knowledge, the means of acquisition, and its validity in the world guide practitioners' approaches in designing and conducting qualitative research. While theoretical assumptions are not always made explicit in published research, "they nonetheless frame the kinds of questions researchers decide to ask, how they go about answering them, and how debates about the soundness of their findings are conducted" (Green & Thorogood, 2004, p. 6).

THEORETICAL PERSPECTIVES IN QUALITATIVE RESEARCH

Theoretical perspectives considered central to qualitative research range from macro (large-scale) theories about the world to middle-range theories, which in turn link to epistemologic theories about the type of knowledge that should be produced through research. The qualitative researcher's theoretical and epistemologic orientation will influence the research questions addressed in a study as well as the methods chosen to address them. A selection rather than an exhaustive list of methodologic orientations commonly employed in qualitative enquiry, including those that may have utility in clinical trials, are briefly described.

Ethnography

Culture is the central focus of ethnographic theory and methodology. Early 20th century anthropologic studies investigated distant and exotic cultures of the 'primitive' world to explore their patterns of living, values, beliefs, and everyday actions. By the middle of the 20th century, ethnography had become a prominent means by which to understand hidden and 'deviant' subcultures in Western society, such as those of street gangs and drug users (Liamputtong, 2009). Medical anthropology uses ethnography to understand health beliefs and healing systems.

Ethnographers tend to use fieldwork methods such as participant observation, indepth interviews, focus groups, and life histories, all of which provide opportunity for extensive and prolonged interaction with research participants. These methods can provide rich data from which the researcher develops the 'thick description' that characterizes the ethnographic account (or research report). Ethnography might also be used as a precursor to other research work. For example, a brief ethnographic study of clinical sites may be used to explore barriers to random allocation in a large clinical trial (Green & Thorogood, 2004).

Phenomenology

This theoretical perspective aims to generate knowledge about how research participants subjectively experience phenomena, often referred to as the 'lived experience' (Daly, 2007). The phenomenologist may be interested in questions such as how an individual experiences a mental illness. Any prejudgements about that reality must be suspended, so that the researcher can "understand and describe the participants' experiences of their everyday world as they see it" (Daly, 2007, p. 98). Phenomenologists employ a range of qualitative methods to gather data for analysis, including indepth interviews, life histories, narratives, observations, diaries, journals, and artworks such as drawings, poetry, and music (Liamputtong, 2009).

Postmodernism

Postmodernist researchers reject the notion that there exists a single reality or truth (Angrosino, 2007; Liamputtong, 2009). Positing that, "realities are constructed within a specific social and cultural context" (Liamputtong, 2009, p. 10), postmodernists deconstruct the meanings held by research participants as well as the language participants use, in order to emphasize the plurality of experience. All stories and expressions of those stories are considered legitimate, and no one story or experience is privileged over others. The aim is to consider society "as a series of fragments in continuous flux" (Liamputtong, 2009, p. 10), and to present and understand each fragment in its own right, rather than as part of a paradigmatic whole.

Along with new epistemologic and methodologic practices, postmodernist researchers have developed innovative methods for collecting data, including arts-based enquiry, online research, and autoethnography, which in recent decades has had much influence on the qualitative research tradition as well as the ways in which researchers write about their work (Liamputtong & Rumbold, 2008; Richardson, 1997, 1999, 2002).

Hermeneutics

The aim of hermeneutics, also known as 'hermeneutic phenomenology' and 'interpretive phenomenology', is to understand human action within context. There are many forms of hermeneutics but two common features of this approach are that (1) language is the essence of all understanding and (2) context (historical context, in particular) provides the framework for such understanding (Willis, 2007).

Due to this focus on language as a precondition for understanding, texts are the very foundation of data in hermeneutics. These may include texts in published materials such as newspapers, journals and blogs, government reports, policy papers, and the like, as well as private documents such as diaries, narratives, memoirs, and personal accounts.

Middle-Range Theories

Middle-range theories provide a link from the broad, abstract theory underpinning the research to observable behavior in everyday contexts (Green & Thorogood, 2004). They are often embedded in particular disciplines and provide explanatory models from which possible research questions might be derived. Table 6.1 provides examples of how a mid-range theory might suggest relevant research questions that can be answered using different methods of collecting and analyzing data.

Table 6.1 Application of Different Methods of Collecting and Analyzing Data in Mid-Range Theory

Middle-Range Theory	Research Question/Aim	Methods of Data Collection	Analysis
Lack of compliance reflects a failure in the clinical trial protocol	Are clinical trial participants more likely to comply with their assigned treatment regimen if they have an opportunity to discuss their concerns with a health professional?	Indepth interviews Observation Clinical notes	Discourse analysis Interpretive thematic analysis Semiotic analysis
The likelihood of a person engaging in a particular behavior depends on her or his assessment of the costs and benefits of that behavior as well as the person's perception of her or his vulnerability to illness (*health belief model*, Becker, 1974)	What risks and benefits do patients associate with participation in clinical trials?	Autoethnographical accounts Focus groups Interviews	Narrative analysis Case study analysis Grounded theory Thematic analysis
Incongruence between the cultural models of mental illness held by patients and by clinicians is a barrier to effective health communication	To explore cultural models of clinical trial participants and staff	Indepth interviews Focus groups	Domain analysis Case study analysis
Lay perceptions of medication risks and benefits differ from those of health professionals	What sources of knowledge do patients draw upon to assess the risks and benefits of medications? How do patients and health professionals explain risks and benefits?	Clinical observation Interviews Focus groups Questionnaire	Interpretive thematic analysis Discourse analysis Semiotic analysis Content analysis

Sources: Green and Thorogood (2004) and Liamputtong (2009).

MIXED METHODS RESEARCH DEFINED

"Mixed methods research is the type of research in which a researcher or team of researchers combines elements of qualitative and quantitative research approaches (e.g., use of qualitative and quantitative viewpoints, data collection, analysis, inference techniques) for the broad purposes of breadth and depth of understanding and corroboration" (Johnson, Onwuegbuzie, & Turner, 2007).

Using a mixed-methods approach within clinical trials may increase the potential to detect meaningful patterns and other phenomena that might otherwise be missed. Triangulation is the use of more than one method to add breadth and depth to data and their analysis, thus contributing to a greater confidence in findings (Bryman, Bell, & Teevan, 2009; Halcomb & Andrew, 2005). Beyond triangulation, mixed-methods designs build on the strengths of different approaches; for example, quantitative methods allow for larger sample sizes, examination of trends and permit generalizability, whereas smaller sample sizes with qualitative methods enable indepth examination of data.

As Creswell, Fetters, and Ivankova (2004) note, "This form of research is more than simply collecting both quantitative and qualitative data; it indicates that data will be integrated, related, or mixed at some stage of the research process. The underlying logic of mixing is that neither quantitative nor qualitative methods are sufficient in themselves to capture the trends and details of the situation. When used in combination, both quantitative and qualitative data yield a more complete analysis, and they complement each other."

A wide variety of designs in mixed methods for health research have been described, typically ascribing greater or lesser weight to either the qualitative or quantitative components of the research, as dictated by the study objectives. For example, Morgan (1998) delineated four complementary mixed methods designs that describe the sequencing of the qualitative and quantitative study phases (i.e., (1) preliminary qualitative methods in a quantitative study; (2) preliminary quantitative methods in a qualitative study; (3) follow-up qualitative methods in a quantitative study (most clinical trial studies will fall in this category); and (4) follow-up quantitative methods in a qualitative study). When using mixed-method designs, it is particularly important to be transparent in terms of reporting the rationale for the selected design. Useful reporting frameworks and recommendations for visualization diagrams are provided in key mixed-methods textbooks (e.g., Creswell & Plano Clark, 2007).

USING QUALITATIVE METHODOLOGIES IN CLINICAL TRIALS

As alluded to above, methodologic orientations in qualitative research speak to theoretical orientations. The four qualitative methodologies introduced in this chapter may have greater or lesser utility in the design of clinical trials, depending on specific study objectives. It is not difficult to see how important it is for the researcher to identify and understand the theoretical assumptions underpinning the study prior to incorporating a qualitative methodology into its design. In the following section, we use a hermeneutic framework to illustrate how a qualitative methodology might be used to maximize the outcomes of a clinical trial.

Research Strategy

Suppose a clinical trial is to be conducted to confirm and further explore a specific clinical syndrome's response to an agent of interest. The researchers decide to incorporate qualitative methods in order to meet the exploratory objective of the study.

Even in cases in which the qualitative arm of a study is purely exploratory in nature, it is important to identify and articulate (broadly) what the study needs to find out. "Knowing what you want to find out leads inexorably to the question of how you will get that information" (Miles & Huberman, 1984, p. 42). Given that enormous quantities of data can be generated from qualitative research with relatively small participant samples, focusing the research will help to avoid collecting data that may be superfluous to the aims of the study. This strategy includes, for example, identifying orienting questions and distinguishing them from focused and open questions. Will the emphasis be on comparison of data (e.g., cross-case comparison), more so than depth (case study)? Cross-case comparison will be aided by having a larger sample size than is needed for an indepth case study, and will benefit from inclusion of standardized research instruments (Silverman & Marvasti, 2008), such as questionnaires and interview topic guides. Predefining the study's methods and measures in this way will help to focus the study's objectives.

Research Methods

In qualitative research, there is no right or wrong method, only methods appropriate to the study and its aims. However, it is important to remember that methods are linked to both methodology and to society. Indeed, "methods are techniques that take on a specific meaning according to the methodology in which they are used" (Silverman & Marvasti, 2008, p. 145). For this reason, researchers need to avoid treating research methods as "mere *techniques*" (Silverman & Marvasti, 2008, p. 145). The hermeneutic approach of our hypothetical study involves methods that use language (verbal or written) to understand and interpret participants' experience in the context of a clinical trial. Opportunities for participants to respond to both focused and open-ended questions about their experience at points in the clinical trial would, therefore, be optimal. Brief interviews, indepth interviews, and questionnaires are methods that lend themselves to collection of this type of data.

Transcripts from audio recordings may provide the primary data source (designated clinical encounters may be recorded in their entirety, or clinicians and participants may record their observations separately following a clinical visit) supplemented by brief case notes and clinical measures taken during the clinical encounter. Questionnaires or topic guides may be used to provide a focus for discussion during the clinical encounter, or the encounter may be entirely free flowing apart from the recording of measures needed for the clinical trial arm of the study. Alternatively, or in addition, clinician researcher observation, clinician researcher case notes, and participant notes could also provide rich sources of data. The case notes may be written during and/or after every clinical encounter, at designated clinical encounters (e.g., first, third, and final visit), or at time intervals (study commencement, 3 months, 6 months, 18 months) regardless of the number of clinical visits. Clinician observation and participant notes may be written responses to focused or open-ended questions provided in a printed questionnaire, at a computer terminal, or online in a secured environment.

The study's researchers and clinicians will need to collaborate in deciding upon the best and most practical methods by which to achieve the study's aims while optimizing both clinician and participant responses. Which methods and what format will provide sufficient detail from clinician researcher observations and notes while avoiding the task becoming onerous over what is likely to be an extended period of time? Scant or truncated clinician notes may provide little data of value to the study's aims. How might participants be prompted to provide sufficient information about their experience so as to be of value to the study? Some participants may provide very little information when they are experiencing positive results or alternatively too much when they are not, or vice versa. Another consideration is how to interpret participant responses; this is important in design of both data collection and data analysis.

Other considerations include the physical, social, and organizational contexts in which participants are to provide their responses. For example, it may be prudent to consult the literature on how people talk with health professionals and each other in contrast to how they respond to researchers' questions in a clinical context (Silverman & Marvasti, 2008), as this may influence the way in which the data are to be collected.

Sampling and Analysis

The sample size will be determined by the aim of the study. Since the study is to be conducted as part of, and in parallel with, a clinical trial, probability sampling is likely to be the dominant strategy. From this, the researchers may decide to use purposive sampling for a case study, thereby explicitly selecting interviewees most likely to be able to provide rich information on the focal research topic. In addition, or alternatively, they may use a theoretical sampling method, continuing to sample and analyze data until no new themes are generated, known as 'sampling to saturation' (Green & Thorogood, 2004; Strauss & Corbin, 1990).

"Analysis of qualitative data relies on both rigour and imagination" (Green & Thorogood, 2004, p. 173). In medical and health research in particular, transparency in reporting methods of analysis is important in ensuring that the researchers' interpretations of the data are credible and that links between the data and those interpretations are clear.

In our hypothetical study, we have chosen the theoretical sampling method, which comes from grounded theory, an open-ended approach developed by American sociologists Barney Glaser and Anselm Strauss (1967) and based on hermeneutics (Huston, 1998). The strength of this approach lies in its circular nature, in which data are collected, analyzed, and coded according to a provisional coding scheme, then used to further sample, analyze, and code data to the point of saturation (Green & Thorogood, 2004). Grounded theory techniques for open coding, identifying emerging theory, and subsequent coding and analysis are described elsewhere (Glaser & Strauss, 1967; Green & Thorogood, 2004; Strauss, 1987).

In coding and analyzing the data, potential categories of interest in our clinical trial may include improvement or worsening in particular clinical features, or persistence, consequent burden, or lack of change in an aspect of a person's mental state and so on. The focus of this method is on the identification and extrapolation of those thematic constructs that determine the clinical denominators for the categories of clinical change. For example, in a previous study using this method (Berk *et al.*, 2010), two classes of data were distilled: transitions (essentially, improvements) in key mental state parameters, and persistent or enduring problematic mental state phenomena. These twin themes are indicative of clinically evident changes in mental state, namely improvement, persistence, or worsening of observed clinical features among trial participants. However, this method is not confined to identifying the presence or absence of diagnostic psychiatric features, as implied by pretreatment symptomatic patterns. Rather, transitions in mental state phenomena may be broadly explored through analysis of the qualitative data collected in the study.

Other Materials and Methods

The recruitment of participants and general conduct of the study, including ethics approval and the storage of data, will be determined by the primary study design, in this case the clinical trial.

To aid in the coding and analysis of data, transcripts, notes, and other textual/graphic data may be imported into a computer software program such as Atlas.ti®, MAXqda®, and NVivo®, which are designed to assist in computer-aided qualitative data analysis (CAQDAS) and support a range of methodologic approaches (Bazeley, 2007). However, while CAQDAS can be tremendously time-saving devices, they cannot guard against human error, neither can they be considered a substitute for the sophisticated interpretive tasks required of the skilled qualitative researcher (Otmar, 2012). CAQDAS can be particularly useful for thematic analysis, grounded theory, and content analysis, the latter of which involves quantification of qualitative data (Silverman & Marvasti, 2008). One advantage of using CAQDAS in mixed-methods analysis is that codes and themes emerging from the qualitative data may be linked to psychiatric phenomenology, including operational definitions such as Diagnostic and Statistical Manual of Mental Disorders (DSM) criteria for mental disorders, as well as functional or other outcomes of interest.

AN EXAMPLE: *N*-ACETYLCYSTEINE IN SCHIZOPHRENIA

In the design of a placebo-controlled clinical trial of *N*-acetylcysteine (NAC) for the adjunctive treatment of schizophrenia, qualitative analysis of clinical observational data was integrated into the study. In this research, Berk and colleagues (2010) sought to extend the study's potential by examining a rich but underutilized qualitative dataset. In essence, the addition of a qualitative analysis enabled the researchers to replicate the principal findings of the clinical trial, thereby providing a methodological triangulation that further strengthened those findings. A further benefit was that analysis of the qualitative data highlighted additional significant differences between NAC and placebo-treated patients, particularly with regard to benefits in positive and affective symptoms that were not detected in the clinical trial.

The primary data sources included clinical notes and reports of observations taken by researcher clinicians during clinical visits by participants from both the treatment and placebo groups. The data were imported into NVivo (Version 2, QSR International, Australia) for coding and analysis. Interpretation of codes was based on psychiatric phenomenology and operational definitions stipulated by DSM diagnostic criteria, with particular relevance to schizophrenia.

In coding and analysis of the data, initially several codes were extracted from the textual information and tentatively identified as patterns of discussion, or narrative salience, and later these were analyzed as the overarching themes emerging from the data, as follows. The first step involved screening (combing) of the texts to identify potential themes that defined improvements (transitions) or persistence in mental-state parameters. From the emergent themes identified, the individual codes were then examined for their presence across the full dataset. The next step was a sentence-by-sentence coding of the textual data into the previously defined emergent mental state transitions, which were then recorded. Coding and recoding of the text were undertaken, until the saturation point was attained. At this point, a qualitative salience matrix was generated within the program in which all cases were tabulated by code and theme, thereby providing a frequency salience. After the themes were identified for each individual case, and pooled, the sample was split into the NAC-treated and placebo-treated groups. Finally, a conventional statistical analysis was performed to determine the between-group significance of the individual themes.

The analysis identified two dichotomous thematic constructs that captured the key categories of clinical phenomena: transitions (or improvements) in mental state parameters, and persistent or worsening mental state phenomena. These themes reflected either improvement, or persistence or aggravation of those features among study participants. The methodology employed in the study allowed for the detection of more transitions or improvements in social interaction, insight, self-care, motivation and volition, psychomotor stability and mood reactivity, and euthymia in NAC-treated than placebo-treated participants. Unchanged or persistent clinical features were more commonly seen in the placebo group, including auditory hallucinations, grandiosity, social withdrawal, ideas of reference, and dysthymia (Table 6.2). While this methodology

Table 6.2 N-Acetyl Cysteine (NAC) in Schizophrenia

Themes	Number of Transition NAC	Number of Transition Placebo	P Value[*]
Transitions in Mental State			
1. Improved insight	62	21	**0.000**
2. Adequate self care	81	29	**0.000**
3. Diminished perceptual abnormalities	15	14	0.513
4. Reduction in self harm thoughts	3	1	0.083
5. Improved social interactivity	57	31	**0.007**
6. Motivation and volition	86	19	**0.000**
7. Thought re-organization	17	8	0.054
8. Mood reactivity and euthymia	38	19	**0.013**
9. Psychomotor stability	21	8	**0.023**
10. Diminished delusional thoughts	23	8	0.051
Unchanged Parameters			
1. Dysthymia	24	59	**0.029**
2. Affective flattening	4	14	0.059
3. Auditory hallucinations	51	101	**0.021**
4. Impaired insight	14	24	0.367
5. Self-neglect and poor hygiene	5	15	0.052
6. Social withdrawal	12	32	**0.023**
7. Paranoia or delusions	81	117	0.331
8. Avolition and apathy	16	17	0.810
9. Ideations of reference	13	72	**0.001**
10. Poverty of speech and thoughts	0	3	0.083
11. Grandiosity	6	72	**0.000**
12. Visual hallucinations	9	25	0.146

Source: Adapted with permission, Berk et al. (2010).
[*]Wilcoxon Signed Ranks Test. Bold values are significant.

confirmed the broad pattern of efficacy seen with quantitative analysis, particularly with regard to negative symptoms, many new signals emerged that inspired follow-up studies in bipolar disorder and depression.

BENEFITS AND LIMITATIONS IN USING MIXED METHODS IN CLINICAL TRIALS

There are many examples in the literature of the use of qualitative methodologies to examine the efficacy of pharmacologic therapies (e.g., Munoz-Plaza, Strauss & Astone-Twerell, 2008; Salter *et al.*, 2008). Qualitative methodologies have also been used to gain insight into the subjective experience of participants using study therapies (Chalmers *et al.*, 2007; Phillips & McCann, 2007), as well as their lived experience of the disorders themselves (Mason, Rice & Records, 2005; Michalak *et al.*, 2012). Qualitative methodologies lend themselves in particular to the exploration of patients' subjective experiences, including adherence and acceptance of therapies (Hansen, Tulinius & Hansen, 2007; Verbeek-Heida & Mathot, 2006; Vervoort *et al.*, 2007). There are examples of the use of qualitative methods in the context of randomized designs, but qualitative methods are not yet widely used in the study of pharmacologic agents on illness symptoms (Fitzsimons *et al.*, 2008; Murphy *et al.*, 2005; Murtagh *et al.*, 2007). Mixed-methods research is more frequently used in health services research, where its utility is influenced by pragmatic considerations and the potential limitations of sole reliance on quantitative methods in capturing the complexity of research in healthcare settings (O'Cathain, Murphy & Nicholl, 2007).

The integration and use of qualitative methodologies in clinical trials specifically has its own potential limitations. One might question whether integration is indeed possible, given the inherent differences between qualitative and quantitative approaches. Interpreting textual data and providing purposeful samples are very different from calculating numerical data. The literature rightly suggests caution when analyzing qualitative and quantitative data together, and thorough consideration of the principles of meta-analysis and an ability to deal with contradictory findings (Malterud, 2001).

Rigorous qualitative analysis is highly dependent on the quality of the source data; a rich data source is one that is sufficiently detailed and complete in order to provide a 'thick' description that is both comprehensive and interpretative. The ability to gather rich source data, in turn, relies upon the skill of the qualitative researcher in eliciting such data, including (for instance) obtaining detailed and relevant information from interview and focus group participants.

Qualitative research is often criticized for its reliance on description and interpretation, two of its very strengths. Another criticism is a lack of generalizability; this, too, is not a major concern given that indepth examination of subjective experience is more important in qualitative research than its quantification. Due to space limitations, we are unable to give this topic its deserved consideration. Suffice to note that in recent years many researchers have shown the potential for generalizability of certain types of qualitative findings. As a telling example, Liamputtong (2009, p. 143) and others have asserted that "[i]f … a given experience is possible, it is also subject to universalisation."

A major strength of the use of qualitative methods in clinical trials is that qualitative research is not constrained by the need to have an a-priori hypothesis and corresponding measure. As a consequence, qualitative methods offer the potential to generate unexpected signals from latent associations in the data, possibly leading to discovery of serendipitous clinical effects. Qualitative methods, therefore, are optimized for hypothesis generation rather than hypothesis testing.

The incorporation of qualitative methods into rigorous, placebo-controlled randomized designs adds a further level of insight into the profile of a potential psychotropic agent. This adds the capacity for combining hypothesis-generation methodologies with traditional hypothesis-testing methodologies. The value of this method is likely to be greatest in early-phase clinical trials, when there is typically only an opaque understanding of the potential profile of a novel agent.

CONCLUSION

In this chapter, we explored the use of qualitative methodologies to extending the potential value of clinical trials. We demonstrated how clinical trial methodologies might be usefully augmented with research methods that are hypothesis-generating, able to detect covert, or latent, factors that might emerge in the conduct of a clinical trial and provide indepth understanding of phenomena, including behaviors. Mixed-methods research, referred to by some as the 'third wave' (Johnson & Onwuegbuzie, 2004) of research paradigms after quantitative and qualitative approaches, offers the potential to broaden the otherwise narrow lens of understanding afforded by clinical trials. We argue here that this represents a missed opportunity in clinical trials settings, and that great attention to the incorporation of qualitative methods into clinical trials is warranted.

CONFLICTS OF INTEREST STATEMENT

Michael Berk has received grant/research support from the National Institutes of Health (NIH), Cooperative Research Centre, Simons Autism Foundation, Cancer Council of Victoria, Stanley Medical Research Foundation, MBF, National Health and Medical Research Council (NHMRC), Beyond Blue, Rotary Health, Geelong Medical Research Foundation, Bristol Myers Squibb, Eli Lilly, GlaxoSmithKline, Meat and Livestock Board, Organon, Novartis, Mayne Pharma, Servier, and Woolworths. He has been a speaker for Astra Zeneca, Bristol Myers Squibb, Eli Lilly, GlaxoSmithKline, Janssen Cilag, Lundbeck, Merck, Pfizer, Sanofi Synthélabo, Servier, Solvay, and Wyeth, and served as a consultant to Astra Zeneca,

Bristol Myers Squibb, Eli Lilly, GlaxoSmithKline, Janssen Cilag, Lundbeck Merck, and Servier.

Erin Michalak has received grant/research support from the Canadian Institutes of Health Research, Healthy Minds, Coast Capital Depression Research, and has served as a consultant to Lundbeck.

REFERENCES

Angrosino, M. (2007). *Doing ethnographic and observation research*. London: Sage Publications.

Bazeley, P. (2007). *Qualitative data analysis with NVivo*. London: Sage Publications.

Becker, M. H. (1974). The health belief model and personal health behavior. *Health Education Monographs, 2*, 324–508.

Berk, M., Munib, A., Dean, O., et al. (2010). Qualitative methods in early-phase drug trials: Broadening the scope of data and methods from an RCT of *N*-acetylcysteine in schizophrenia. *Journal of Clinical Psychiatry, 72*, 909–913.

Bryman, A., Bell, E. A., & Teevan, J. J. (2009). *Social research methods* (2nd ed.). New York: Oxford University Press.

Chalmers, A., Mitchell, C., Rosenthal, M., et al. (2007). An exploration of patients' memories and experiences of hyperbaric oxygen therapy in a multiplace chamber. *Journal of Clinical Nursing, 16*, 1454–1459.

Creswell, J. W., Fetters, M. D., & Ivankova, N. V. (2004). Designing a mixed methods study in primary care. *Annals of Family Medicine, 2*, 7–12.

Creswell, J. W., & Plano Clark, V. L. (2007). *Designing and conducting mixed methods research*. Thousand Oaks, CA: Sage Publications.

Daly, K. J. (2007). *Qualitative methods for family studies and human development*. Thousand Oaks, CA: Sage Publications.

Fitzsimons, C. F., Baker, G., Wright, A., et al. (2008). The 'Walking for Wellbeing in the West' randomised controlled trial of a pedometer-based walking programme in combination with physical activity consultation with 12 month follow-up: Rationale and study design. *BMC Public Health, 8*, 259.

Glaser, B., & Strauss, A. (1967). *The discovery of grounded theory: Strategies for qualitative research*. Chicago: Aldine.

Green, J., & Thorogood, N. (2004). *Qualitative methods for health research*. London: Sage Publications.

Halcomb, E. J., & Andrew, S. (2005). Triangulation as a method for contemporary nursing research. *Nurse Researcher, 13*, 71–82.

Hansen, D. L., Tulinius, D., & Hansen, E. H. (2007). Adolescents' struggles with swallowing tablets: Barriers, strategies and learning. *Pharmacy World & Science, 30*, 65–69.

Huston, P. (1998). Qualitative studies: Their role in medical research. *Canadian Family Physician, 44*, 2453–2458.

Hyman, S. E. (2012). Revolution stalled. *Science Translational Medicine, 4*(155), 155.

Johnson, R. B., & Onwuegbuzie, A. J. (2004). Mixed methods research: A research paradigm whose time has come. *Educational Researcher, 33*, 14–26.

Johnson, R. B., Onwuegbuzie, A. J., & Turner, L. A. (2007). Toward a definition of mixed methods research. *Journal of Mixed Methods Research, 1*, 112.

Liamputtong, P. (2009). *Qualitative research methods* (3rd ed.). South Melbourne: Oxford University Press.

Liamputtong, P., & Rumbold, J. (2008). *Knowing differently: Arts-based and collaborative research methods*. New York: Nova Science Publishers.

Malterud, K. (2001). Qualitative research: Standards, challenges, and guidelines. *Lancet, 358*, 483–488.

Mason, W. A., Rice, M. J., & Records, K. (2005). The lived experience of postpartum depression in a psychiatric population. *Perspectives in Psychiatric Care, 41*, 52–61.

Michalak, E. E., Hole, R., Holmes, C., et al. (2012). 'Recovery is such a huge word': Understandings of 'recovery' in people with bipolar disorder and implications for psychiatric care. *Psychiatric Annals*, *42*, 173–178.

Miles, M., & Huberman, A. (1984). *Qualitative data analysis* (2nd ed.). Thousand Oaks, CA: Sage Publications.

Morgan, D. L. (1998). Practical strategies for combining qualitative and quantitative methods: Applications to health research. *Qualitative Health Research*, *8*, 362–376.

Munoz-Plaza, C. E., Strauss, S., & Astone-Twerell, J. (2008). Exploring drug users' attitudes and decisions regarding hepatitis C (HCV) treatment in the U.S. *International Journal of Drug Policy*, *19*, 71–78.

Murphy, A. W., Cupples, M. E., Smith, S. M., et al. (2005). The SPHERE study. Secondary prevention of heart disease in general practice: Protocol of a randomised controlled trial of tailored practice and patient care plans with parallel qualitative, economic and policy analyses. *Current Controlled Trials in Cardiovascular Medicine*, *6*, 11.

Murtagh, M. J., Thomson, R. G., May, C. R., et al. (2007). Qualitative methods in a randomised controlled trial: The role of an integrated qualitative process evaluation in providing evidence to discontinue the intervention in one arm of a trial of a decision support tool. *Quality Safety in Health Care*, *16*, 224–229.

O'Cathain, A., Murphy, E., & Nicholl, J. (2007). Why, and how, mixed methods research is undertaken in health services research in England: A mixed methods study. *BMC Health Services Research*, *7*, 85.

Otmar, R. (2012). Barriers and enablers in the treatment and prevention of osteoporosis: Exploring knowledge, beliefs, attitudes and cultural models among consumers and medical practitioners, Ph.D. thesis. Australia: University of Melbourne.

Phillips, L., & McCann, E. (2007). The subjective experiences of people who regularly receive depot neuroleptic medication in the community. *Journal of Psychiatric and Mental Health Nursing*, *14*, 578–586.

Richardson, L. (1997). *Fields of play: Constructing an academic life*. New Brunswick, NJ: Rutgers University Press.

Richardson, L. (1999). Jeopardy. Paper presented at the Forum Lecture Series, 4 February. Las Vegas: University of Nevada.

Richardson, L. (2002). Poetic representation of interviews. In J. F. Gubrium & J. A. Holstein (Eds.), *Handbook of interview research: Context & method*. Thousand Oaks, CA: Sage Publications.

Salter, M. L., Go, V. F., Celentano, D. D., et al. (2008). The role of men in women's acceptance of an intravaginal gel in a randomized clinical trial in Blantyre, Malawi: A qualitative and quantitative analysis. *AIDS Care*, *20*, 853–862.

Silverman, D., & Marvasti, A. (2008). *Doing qualitative research: A comprehensive guide*. Thousand Oaks, CA: Sage Publications.

Strauss, A. (1987). *Qualitative analysis for social scientists*. Cambridge: Cambridge University Press.

Strauss, A., & Corbin, J. (1990). *Basics of qualitative research: Grounded theory procedures and techniques*. Newbury Park, CA: Sage Publications.

Verbeek-Heida, P. M., & Mathot, E. F. (2006). Better safe than sorry – why patients prefer to stop using selective serotonin reuptake inhibitor (SSRI) antidepressants but are afraid to do so: Results of a qualitative study. *Chronic Illness*, *2*, 133–142.

Vervoort, S. C., Borleffs, J. C., Hoepelman, A. I., et al. (2007). Adherence in antiretroviral therapy: A review of qualitative studies. *AIDS*, *21*, 271–281.

Willis, J. W. (2007). *Foundations of qualitative research: Interpretive and critical approaches*. Thousand Oaks, CA: Sage Publications.

Chapter Seven

Sequential Multiple Assignment Randomized Treatment (SMART): Designs in Bipolar Disorder Clinical Trials

Charles L. Bowden and Vivek Singh

University of Texas Health Science Center at San Antonio, San Antonio, TX, USA

CHAPTER OUTLINE

Clinical Trial Design Challenges in Mood Disorders. DOI: http://dx.doi.org/10.1016/B978-0-12-405170-6.00007-5

INTRODUCTION

The predominant maintenance clinical trial design in all psychiatric treatment studies, as well as many other chronic medical illnesses, involves randomization at the time of enrollment to one of two or three treatment groups: a standard, established comparator, the drug of interest, or placebo. If *any* of the options is unacceptable to the patient, the patient is either excluded from the study or will choose not to enter. Several factors account for a patient's unwillingness to participate in a study or being excluded from participation in the study. Patient-experienced factors include having had adverse effects while taking one of the treatment options or having not experienced any benefit from one of the treatment options. Additionally, a patient may be unwilling to risk one of the adverse effects described as frequently caused by one of the treatment options. Patients may also choose not to take part in the study due to the potential of being randomized to receive placebo. These same factors may contribute to study staff not offering participation to a patient who otherwise qualifies for the study. A third set of factors are ones designated as excluding factors, for example, having made a suicide attempt or having suicidal ideation, having concurrent medical conditions, pregnancy, potential for pregnancy, or out of age range status. The net consequence is that over half of all people with the disorder and clinical disease state of focus are excluded from participation (Bowden *et al.*, 1997).

Traditional maintenance studies are characterized by low generalizability, biases that favor the drug of interest of the funding pharmaceutical corporation and limited relevance to front line clinical practices for illnesses such as bipolar disorder (BD). Most pharmaceutical company-funded studies employ efficacy designs that prioritize internal validity (assay sensitivity) at the expense of external validity (generalizability) (Bowden, 2008). However, once efficacy is established, the responsibility to establish generalizability that will be of practical use to psychiatrists and other clinicians generally reside with academic groups applying designs that emphasize external validity with support from public and private funding sources such as National Institute of Mental Health (NIMH), Patient-Centered Outcomes Research Institute (PCORI) or equivalent not-for-profit organizations. In part the objectives of generalizability, wider clinical application of findings, and development of patient-centered evidence can be accomplished by studying more heterogeneous subgroups, that is, patients who may also have anxiety, substance abuse, metabolic burdens (March *et al.*, 2005), thus representing a wider spectrum of illness manifestation. This action serves the aim of correcting for efficacy-based studies that artificially inflate effect size by excluding difficult-to-treat patients; yielding effectiveness studies with more realistic effect sizes. With the current paradigms in place worldwide for conduct of studies of new treatments, the major investments made by pharmaceutical companies provide only a starting data platform for clinicians, healthcare provider systems, and patients with the diseases of interest on which to base clinical practices. Thus, a major challenge for research leaders, regulatory, health policy, for-profit and not-for-profit funding organizations in the field is to determine how best to move forward on this continuum of improved generalizability.

Substantial evidence also indicates that monotherapy regimens are generally less effective than combination regimens for maintenance treatment of BD (Bowden, Schatzberg & Nemeroff, 2001; Geddes *et al.*, 2010). To date, most studies of adjunctive regimens for maintenance have been based on designs enriched in favor of the adjunctive regimen, which usually includes the drug of interest. This intentional bias is usually accomplished by requiring that the patient tolerates and benefits from the principal drug of interest during an open acute phase of the study, and/or that the patient previously was not been responsive to the comparator drug during an acute open phase. Enriched design maintenance treatment studies in BD have generally reported completion rates below 30% (Suppes *et al.*, 2009; Vieta *et al.*, 2008), which further negatively impacts the generalizability of findings.

SMART METHODOLOGIES

The 2000s has seen the development of innovative research design, in particular sequential multiple assignment randomized trials (SMARTs), to address the above problems in both BD and other chronic diseases. We developed SMART methodology to specifically target problems of poor generalizability and external validity in BD maintenance studies (Thorpe *et al.*, 2009). (Note: we use SMART-BD in the remainder of the chapter when referring to the specific SMART methodology that we developed and are currently testing in a BD maintenance trial, and SMART when referring to the family of current and potentially additional designs that have been developed for other diseases.) First explicitly proposed by Lavori and coworkers as relevant to any chronic disease, only since 2000 have early reports of results of such studies appeared, and that principally in websites (Lavori & Dawson, 2008; Lavori, Dawson & Rush, 2000). SMART-BD design adds at least one additional randomization contingent on evidence of (1) intolerability to the first randomized regimen, or (2) development or persistence of an illness component for which there is evidence of lack of response for the treatments available in the first randomization.

SMART chooses subsequent treatments based on patients' current clinical state and response or tolerability to prior treatment during the trial. Such a strategy mimics the adaptive nature of treatment selection that occurs in routine clinical settings, thereby increasing generalizability and relevance to actual clinical practice. Of equal importance is the improved generalizability consequent to allowing a change in the initial randomized regimen during the planned course of treatment. The randomization in the study design allows for causal inference, consequent to elimination of unmeasured confounders associated with opportunistic, unplanned treatment decisions during treatment (Turner *et al.*, 2013).

SMART designs also serve to reduce a problem commonly seen in maintenance studies due to high rates of dropout consequent to lack of/inadequate efficacy or poor tolerability. The SMART accomplishes this with subsequent randomized treatment options that allow continuation of a subject who would have terminated the study if no protocol-defined treatment regimen changes were allowed/required in response to continued symptoms or inadequate tolerability.

SMART approaches enable taking into account the order in which illness components manifest to guide treatment options, rather than considering each component in isolation. This element in the SMART design is consistent with routine clinical care, thereby further enhances the clinical relevance and external validity of study findings. The primary goal of most SMART studies is the development of evidence-based adaptive intervention strategies, which can then be evaluated in a randomized controlled trial.

A SMART design study also allows studying biomarkers in a controlled environment but with wider generalizability than is possible with a single front end randomization. SMART type studies have been described by other names such as stepped-care strategies (Collins, Murphy & Strecher, 2007; Sobell & Sobell, 2000).

SMART STUDY OF PRIMARY LITHIUM OR VALPROATE IN CLINICALLY SYMPTOMATIC BIPOLAR DISORDER COUPLED WITH SECOND-PHASE RANDOMIZATION TO TREATMENTS FOR DEVELOPING OR PERSISTING CLINICALLY SIGNIFICANT DEPRESSION

NIMH Center grants in services and interventions research require a methods development study aimed at advancing designs in ways that improve generalizability, patient centeredness, and/or some aspect of statistical analysis or other innovative component of the study. We describe a study in progress initiated in 2011 as the methods development protocol for our Advanced Center in Interventions and Services Research (MH grant no. P30MH086045). The conceptual theme of the Center is "Personalizing community-based treatment of bipolar disorder to improve outcomes." Specifically relevant to the SMART-BD study, we expected the personalized aspects of the SMART study to increase treatment acceptability, enhance adherence, and outcomes, and reduce disparities. In the grant proposal, we noted that "the adaptive design to be studied may provide a pathway forward for testing of new drugs and methodologies that will break the 50 year pattern of failure to design studies that yield generalizable data and facilitate the development of molecules with novel mechanisms and benefits." The SMART study was expected to comport more closely with effective clinical management of BD, which involves adapting a treatment plan to a patient's current mood state and history, choosing an initial treatment, reassessing the treatment based on efficacy and tolerability, and reiteration of the decision process. The adaptive design was expected to yield more ecologically valid results, addressing the Food and Drug Association (FDA) and public health concerns about biasing associated with current study designs used in registration maintenance studies.

SYNOPSIS OF THE 26-WEEK, OPEN, RANDOMIZED SMART BIPOLAR DISORDER STUDY

Participants

Subjects will be ages 18 years or older with BD I or II and clinically significant symptomatology (Clinical Global Impression – Severity – Bipolar Disorder, CGI-BP-S, 3 or greater for mania/hypomania and/or depression) for 2 weeks or greater.

Study Summary

This two-site, open randomized study will treat 200 patients for 26 weeks with 150 at the University of Texas Health Science Center at San Antonio, TX and 50 at Case Western University, Cleveland, OH. The primary efficacy measure, CGI-BP-S, will be blinded.

Induction Phase

After a washout period of up to 1 week, patients will be openly randomized to treatment with a mood stabilizer (MS), lithium (Li) or divalproex extended release (DV) for at least 2 weeks. Patients who become intolerant to Li or DV at any point through week 22 will be crossed to the other MS and continued in the study.

Maintenance Phase

The maintenance phase is 24 weeks. Patients who respond adequately to either DV or Li at the end of 2 weeks (CGI-BP-S $\leq$ 2 for depression plus tolerability to MS) will be continued on the assigned MS. Patients who have clinically significant depression (CGI-Depression-S $\geq$ 3) for 1 week at any point starting at week 2 through week 20 will additionally be randomized to one of three regimens: MS alone, MS plus quetiapine (QT) (MS + QT) or MS plus lamotrigine (LM) (MS + LM). Patients with a CGI-Depression-S of 3 or greater at week

2 will have an extra visit scheduled for week 3 to determine whether the criteria for the second randomization are met. Treatment will be terminated if a patient has a score of 4 on the Bipolar Inventory of Signs and Symptoms Scale (BISS) – suicide, BISS-depression 50 or greater, or BISS Mania score 35 or greater for 4 consecutive weeks, or if the treating psychiatrist determines that a patient poses an imminent risk of self harm. Patients unable to tolerate Li or DV at minimum therapeutic serum levels of 0.5 mEq/L (or 45 mg/L) will be switched to the alternative MS.

Disposition of Subjects and Sample Size of Groups

Based on published data, we estimate that 90% of enrolled subjects will meet all eligibility criteria and have at least one dose of study medication and 90% of those (162 patients) assigned to initial MS will develop depression within 20 weeks and enter the second randomized group, yielding a total of 54 patients in each of the adjunctive treatment and 70 in the MS alone group, including 18 that will have been continued on DV or Li without having experienced depression.

Medications

Li/DV will be dosed to attain Li or DV levels of 0.5 mEq/L or greater ($\geq$45 g/L). LM will be incrementally dosed up to 400 mg/day, or, in combination with DV, 200 mg/day. Extended release Li or DV are recommended, but timing of dosage and type of formulation are at the discretion of the treating psychiatrist. QT will be started at 50 mg/day and titrated up to 300 mg/day as tolerated. The minimum dosage for QT or LM is 100 mg/day with Li or 50 mg/day with DV. Patients not tolerating the minimal targeted dosage of QT or LM can be continued in the SMART protocol if they agree to take the maximum adequately tolerated dose of QT or LM for the remainder of the study.

Benzodiazepines (lorazepam equivalent of 4 mg/day as needed) will be permitted during the entire course of the study for anxiety, agitation, and irritability. Subjects will be allowed the use of a sleep-inducing agent, zaleplon or zolpidem, 5–10 mg at night as needed for sleep. Trihexyphenidyl, 5 mg twice daily as needed may be prescribed for extrapyramidal adverse effects.

Patients eligible for the study who are taking any second-generation antipsychotic (SGA) other than QT at the time of study entry may continue the drug in the protocol, but with no option to increase the dose. The SGA may be discontinued at any time for perceived adverse effects and if the patient experiences depression as defined previously the SGA must be tapered off over a 1- to 2-week period. The time of discontinuation will start the period for eligibility for the second randomization for depression.

Patients taking any antidepressant may start the study while continuing the antidepressant, and the antidepressant must be discontinued over a 1- to 4-week period, as clinically feasible, with the period of eligibility for second randomization commencing at the time of discontinuation.

Assessments

Assessments are shown in Table 7.1.

Baseline measurements include:

- demographics, the Mini International Neuropsychiatric Interview (MINI);
- medical problem checklist;
- ethnicity/race, language;
- morningness/eveningness;
- discrimination/devaluation;
- insurance costs, patient satisfaction with care;
- laboratory tests: urine pregnancy, thyroid-stimulating hormone (TSH), master chem. Including lipid panel, fasting, complete blood count, serum Li, val. Repeat TSH, chem. If patient has second randomization;
- weight, height (in CPR), waist circumference. Repeat if patient switches MS, or has second randomization and at study end;
- Vital signs: temperature, pulse rate, respiratory rate, blood pressure, and at study end.

Criteria for Recovered Status

Recovered status requires 4 or more consecutive weeks with CGI-BP-S less than 3, BISS Depression score less than 18 and BISS Manic score less than 11.

Hypothesis: A.2.1

Li and DV will not differ in efficacy. Lack of acceptability, defined as (1) discontinuation for adverse effects, (2) developing any adverse effect that rates moderate in severity and persists for 2 weeks or requires treatment will be greater for Li than for DV and will not differ between Hispanic, non-Hispanic white and African-American subjects. Analysis plan: we will look both

Table 7.1 Table of Assessments

Assessments	Q 3 months	All Visits	Rater	Purpose
Baseline: see below				
BISS (5 factors, YMRS, MADRS)	–	X	Research coordinator	Outcome, signs, behavioral domains
CPR: BISS-15, GAF, CGI-S, CGI-D, and CGI-M	–	X	Clinician	Outcome, validity, concordance
BISS-SR includes adherence	–	X	Patient	Outcome, concordance
Life Function Questionnaire	X	–	–	Moderators

BISS: Bipolar Inventory of Signs and Symptoms; BISS-SR: Bipolar Inventory of Signs and Symptoms – Self Rated; CGI-D: Clinical Global Impression – Depression; CGI-M: Clinical Global Impression – Mania; CGI-S: Clinical Global Impression – Severity; GAF: Global Assessment of Functioning; MADRS: Montgomery and Åsberg Depression Rating Scale; YMRS: Young Mania Rating Scale.

at the initial randomization to Li versus DV and the drug after crossover if it occurs (i.e., the maintenance MS) as the basis for analysis. As permitted in most of the proposed analysis methods, current MS (Li, DV) will be included as a time-varying covariate in addition to baseline (randomized) MS. Development of adverse effects will be coded as a dichotomous (yes-no) outcome at each assessment point, and analyzed using a generalized linear mixed effects regression model (i.e., mixed effects logistic regression with repeated measures).

Hypothesis A.3.1

Both MS + QT and MS + LM will be more efficacious than MS alone in subjects who develop depression with no difference between QT and LM. Analysis plan: the hypotheses call for a three-group design in the subsamples that develop depression. The hypotheses call for an omnibus test of overall differences, with planned contrasts comparing MS + QT and MS + LM groups with MS, and comparing the MS + QT and MS + LM groups with each other. We propose reduction in BISS – Depression and improvement in CGI-D within 6 weeks as two primary outcomes and sustained recovery as a secondary measure of efficacy. We will operationalize sustained recovery as time-to-event outcomes and analyze with survival analysis methods.

Supplementary analyses will add consideration of effects of baseline clinical and descriptive confounders, BD I versus BD II, initial and current MS, and time-dependent adjunctive anxiolytic treatment.

Hypothesis A.2.2

LM will be significantly more acceptable than QT. Plan: analyses of acceptability of LM versus QT within the depressed subsample will be done as for the analyses described in 'Hypothesis A.2.1' above.

Hypothesis A.2.3

Subjects receiving QT or LM will show greater improvement over time in symptom domains of BD including depression, mania, and function relative to subjects randomized to MS only. Plan: in addition to the primary outcome, several important dependent measures are listed: major symptom domains (BISS), side effects, and functional capacity.

Exploratory Analyses and Qualitative Aim 1

To determine the effects of ethnicity, language, education, and stress as moderators of treatment outcomes. Explore complexities and operational benefits and difficulties experienced with the SMART. Explore the use of novel statistical methodologies to characterize illness trajectories in response to the interventions more informatively. Plan: to address strengths and limitations of the SMART design we will report descriptive statistics such as recruitment rates, dropout, implementation difficulties, or evidence of site-specific factors.

Power Analyses

The initial randomization of all recruited patients randomizes 90 patients either to Li or DV. With 180 participants, power for survival regression is 0.80 to detect a hazard ratio of 2.0 (e.g., retention rates of 85% vs. 71%; 73% vs. 54%; 65% vs. 42%). Most of the major analyses concern the maintenance sample of 54 patients adjunctively on QT, 54 adjunctively on LM, and 72 on MS alone (with unequal numbers of participants this is an effective sample size of 59). A simple three-group analysis of variance (ANOVA) without repeated measures has power of 0.85 to detect a conventional medium effect of $f = 0.25$. This is a conservative estimate of power for the proposed analyses because use of a baseline covariate and repeated measures both will increase power.

Innovation and Significance

This adaptive design can strengthen inferences about treatment outcomes, particularly for effectiveness. The study allows for greater inclusivity in subject enrollment, enhancing generalizability of findings and emphasizes indices of sustained benefit, rather than basing efficacy on a single point in time assessment. The sample size will support comparisons of Hispanic and African-American subjects with non-Hispanic subjects and subjects in academic settings with those in public sector clinics, thereby contributing to a better understanding of specific features of conduct of intervention research in community settings that determine success or the lack thereof. *The study addresses an important public health question: can clinical trials design incorporate a reasonable level of randomization to be applied over the course of a treatment study for BD in a manner that personalizes treatments and optimizes outcomes and provides evidence based guidelines to clinicians? In other areas of medicine, adaptive designs have yielded novel results; but no published study in BD has compared the merits and limitations of such designs.*

APPROACH AND FEASIBILITY

SMART designs have the potential to yield greater clinically relevant effectiveness results and facilitate development of novel treatments in BD. Monotherapy regimens with first-line treatments for BD are insufficient to avoid high proportions of missing data consequent to early study discontinuation, regardless of investigator or subject intent. LM monotherapy was superior to placebo for BD in maintenance care, principally for depressive relapses but less than 30% of LM-treated patients completed the studies (Geddes, Calabrese & Goodwin, 2009).

CONSIDERATION IN PLANNING AND EXECUTING SMART PROTOCOLS

Despite the numerous advantages that SMART designs can readily provide, the methodology has some important limitations. The number of secondary or tertiary randomization points will limit power, since in most SMART studies intervention points beyond the first one will apply only to a subset of subjects enrolled. Furthermore, the number of people warranting the second or third randomization can only be estimated prior to actual conduct of the study. A related issue is that the duration of exposure to a regimen will vary substantially since subsequent randomization is dependent on either the persistence or development of some component of the illness, which may vary between patients. Additionally, if the protocol allows randomization contingent on patient response without any time limit, the period of assessment of the dynamic intervention could be insufficient to test the hypothesis associated with the second- or third-order intervention.

SMART designs can include a placebo, or monotherapy arm, at a secondary intervention point. For example, in the 26-week study described above, for patients who develop or have sustained clinically significant depression from the time of enrollment, we include a third arm for depressive intervention to be sustained monotherapy with the MS that the patient is taking at the point of intervention for depression.

SELECTIVE REVIEW OF SMART STUDIES IN OTHER AREAS OF MEDICINE

Investigators working in other disease or therapeutic areas are quite enthusiastic regarding adaptive, or sometimes similarly but not identically defined dynamic studies. However, the emphases regarding benefits to be gained, or the specific approaches to achieve the within-study secondary randomized interventions, often differ. Almirall and colleagues, working in the area of social research, notes that "An adaptive intervention is a sequence of individually tailored decisions rules that specify whether, how, and when to alter the intensity, type, or delivery of treatment at critical decision points in the medical care process" (Almirall *et al.*, 2012). Adaptive interventions are particularly well suited for the management of chronic diseases, but can be used in any clinical setting in which sequential medical decision-making is essential for the welfare of the patient. They have potential to enhance clinical outcomes by flexibly tailoring treatments to patients when they need it most, and in the most appropriate dose. Penn State University (State College, PA) maintains a comprehensive array of information on SMART studies, including a list of currently extramurally funded studies, highlighted studies, brief commentaries, and locations and contact information for individuals and groups working in the areas of SMART and other dynamic study designs (http://methodology.psu.edu/; last accessed 29 July 2014). In addition to timely material available from the Penn State University Methodology Center, published studies employing some aspect of SMART methodologies are accessible in the areas of attention deficit hyperactivity disorder (ADHD) treatment (Pelham & Fabiano, 2008), naltrexone treatment for alcoholism (Murphy *et al.*, 2007), contingency management for cocaine dependence (Petry *et al.*, 2012), and prostate cancer (Wang *et al.*, 2012).

Sequential treatments are often required because treatment effects are heterogeneous, with some patient responding well, others not at all, and others partially to the same intervention. Such heterogeneity requires some modulation of the intervention, either addition of a plausibly complementary treatment, a switch in treatment, or, less likely, a dosage change in the initial treatment.

In addition, a treatment that is initially effective for a patient may provide less benefit, or cause more adverse effects over time. In most cases, it is essential to assess benefits of a drug or overall regimen versus the adverse effects of the regimen, an issue that often differs across time. Attention to protocols for sequencing different regimens has received more attention in cancer therapy, plausibly because the short-term tolerability and/or long-term consequences of a regimen are often compromising to quality of life. A particularly comprehensive consideration of such tradeoffs of benefits and adverse effects is incorporated in the report of dynamic treatment regimens in prostate cancer (Wang *et al.*, 2012).

PROSPECTIVE DESIGN CONSIDERATIONS FOR SMART STUDIES

Scientists need evidence that a planned dynamic intervention is viable from the perspective of safety, tolerability, simplicity, and cost and benefits for symptoms viewed as essential for attention by patients and clinicians (Lavori *et al.*, 2000; March *et al.*, 2005). One step in achieving these goals is to be operationally clear on how subsequent treatment options within the SMART are implemented, and earlier interventions terminated or modified. Consideration of common contingencies regarding continuation or termination of an earlier instituted treatment need to be operationally thought through in planning of a study.

A second important step to ensure that the embedded dynamic treatment regimens are viable is a clear, detailed plan of how to treat patients in the event that additional common contingencies (e.g., beyond what is typically thought of as course-specific success or failure) arise during treatment. Such contingencies may include intolerable side effects (e.g., toxicity in the treatment of cancer, or weight gain in the treatment of schizophrenia), excessive treatment burden (such as is possible with preventive and behavioral interventions), and treatment dropout or refusal to receive subsequent treatment (such as may happen with almost any intervention). The clinical trial protocol, including the materials provided to the Data Safety Monitoring Board and/or Institutional Review Boards, can be useful for successfully addressing this objective.

MATCHING THE STATISTICAL ANALYSIS TO THE RATIONALE FOR A SMART

We supply substantial protocol details from our in progress SMART, in part to convey the strategic planning needed regarding statistical analyses. Conducting time-to-event survival analysis is unlikely to assess the acceptability and generalizability of information on each aspect of the SMART study adequately, as well as the overall study objectives (Lei *et al.*, 2012).

REFERENCES

Almirall, D., Compton, S. N., Gunlicks-Stoessel, M., et al. (2012). Designing a pilot sequential multiple assignment randomized trial for developing an adaptive treatment strategy. *Statistics in Medicine, 17,* 1887–1902.

Bowden, C. L. (2008). Bipolar pathophysiology and development of improved treatments: Review and recommendations for innovative studies. *Brain Research, 1235,* 92–97.

Bowden, C. L., Schatzberg, A. F., & Nemeroff, C. B. (2001). *Chapter 18. Treatment of bipolar disorder.* Washington DC: American Psychiatric Publishing Inc. pp. 387–397.

Bowden, C. L., Swann, A. C., Calabrese, J. R., et al. (1997). Maintenance clinical trials in bipolar disorder: Design implications of the divalproex-lithium-placebo study. *Psychopharmacology Bulletin, 33,* 693–699.

Collins, L. M., Murphy, S. A., & Strecher, V. (2007). The Multiphase Optimization Strategy (MOST) and the Sequential Multiple Assignment Randomized Trial (SMART). New methods for more potent ehealth interventions. *American Journal of Preventive Medicine, 32,* S112–S118.

Geddes, J. R., Calabrese, J. R., & Goodwin, G. M. (2009). Lamotrigine for treatment of bipolar depression: Independent meta-analysis and meta-regression of individual patient data from five randomised trials. *British Journal of Psychiatry, 194,* 4–9.

Geddes, J. R., Goodwin, G. M., Rendell, J., et al. (2010). Lithium plus valproate combination therapy versus monotherapy for relapse prevention in bipolar I disorder (BALANCE): A randomised open-label trial. *Lancet, 375,* 385–395.

Lavori, P. W., & Dawson, R. (2008). Adaptive treatment strategies in chronic disease. *Annual Review of Medicine, 59,* 443–453.

Lavori, P. W., Dawson, R., & Rush, A. J. (2000). Flexible treatment strategies in chronic disease: Clinical and research implications. *Biological Psychiatry, 48,* 605–614.

Lei, H., Nahum-Shani, I., Lynch, K., et al. (2012). A "SMART" design for building individualized treatment sequences. *Annual Review of Clinical Psychology, 8,* 21–48.

March, J. S., Silva, S. G., Compton, S., et al. (2005). The case for practical clinical trials in psychiatry. *American Journal of Psychiatry, 162,* 836–846.

Murphy, S. A., Lynch, K. G., Oslin, D. W., et al. (2007). Developing adaptive treatment strategies in substance abuse research. *Drug Alcohol Dependence, 88,* S24–S30.

Pelham, W. E., & Fabiano, G. A. (2008). Evidence-based psychosocial treatment for ADHD: An update. *Journal of Clinical Child and Adolescent Psychology, 31,* 184–214.

Petry, N. M., Barry, D., Alessi, S. M., et al. (2012). A randomized trial adapting contingency management targets based on initial abstinence status of cocaine-dependent patients. *Journal of Consulting and Clinical Psychology, 80,* 276–285.

Sobell, M. B., & Sobell, S. L. (2000). Stepped care as a heuristic approach to the treatment of alcohol problems. *Journal of Consulting Clinical Psychology, 68,* 573–579.

Suppes, T., Vieta, E., Liu, S., et al. (2009). Maintenance treatments for patients with bipolar I disorder: Results from a North American study of quetiapine in combination with lithium or divalproex (trial 127). *American Journal of Psychiatry, 166,* 476–488.

Thorpe, K. E., Zwarenstein, M., Oxman, A. D., et al. (2009). A pragmatic explanatory continuum indicator summary (PRECIS): A tool to help trial designers. *Journal of Clinical Epidemiology, 62,* 464e–475e.

Turner, E. H., Matthews, A. M., Linardatos, E., et al. (2013). Selective publication of antidepressant trials and its influence on apparent efficacy. *New England Journal of Medicine, 358,* 252–260.

Vieta, E., Suppes, T., Eggens, I., et al. (2008). Efficacy and safety of quetiapine in combination with lithium or divalproex for maintenance of patients with bipolar I disorder. *Journal of Affective Disorders, 109,* 251–263.

Wang, L., Rotnitzky, A., Lin, X., et al. (2012). Evaluation of viable dynamic treatment regimes in a sequentially randomized trial of advanced prostate cancer. *Journal of the American Statistical Association, 107,* 493–508.

Chapter | Eight

Novel Study Designs for Clinical Trials in Mood Disorders

Hong Jin Jeon[1,2] and Maurizio Fava[1]

[1]*Harvard Medical School, Boston, MA, USA;*
[2]*Samsung Medical Center, Sungkyunkwan University School of Medicine, Seoul, Korea*

CHAPTER OUTLINE

Clinical Trial Design Challenges in Mood Disorders. DOI: http://dx.doi.org/10.1016/B978-0-12-405170-6.00008-7

INTRODUCTION

The standard double-blind, placebo-controlled trial in mood disorders compares the efficacy of a specific treatment/treatments with that of placebo for subjects identified according to prior criteria. It uses the parallel comparison of one or more treatments with placebo, with sample sizes considered adequate to detect a therapeutic signal, given the expected placebo response rates in that specific population.

'Placebo' is defined as an inactive substance or preparation used as a control in an experiment or test to determine the efficacy of a medicine or treatment. 'Placebo response' is defined as a change that occurs following the administration of a placebo. 'Placebo effect' is a difference between the placebo response and those changes that occur without the administration of a placebo, which is typically never quantified. If a patient showed improvement after given a placebo, there are some questions should be addressed.

1. "Is it the result of the placebo itself?"
2. "Is it due to natural fluctuations in the progression of the disease?"
3. "Is it regression toward the mean?"
4. "Is it due to nonspecific, treatment effects?"
5. "Is it due to patients' and clinicians' expectations?"

As the term is commonly used, placebo response represents an apparent improvement in the clinical condition of mood disorder patients randomly assigned to the placebo treatment (e.g., a pre-post-treatment change within the placebo group). In a mood disorder clinical trial, patients can be classified accordingly to their intrinsic propensity to respond or not to active versus placebo treatment (Figure 8.1). The patients who respond to either drug or placebo (D+P+) are relatively uninformative as they do not show differential responsiveness and therefore cannot detect a signal for a given compound. Patients who respond to placebo but not to drug (D−P+) are relatively uncommon and they represent a negligible proportion of subjects. The only informative group is represented by the patients who respond to drug but not to placebo (D+P−), but the size of such group is affected by the size of the group of patients who are resistant to treatment and therefore show no response to either drug or placebo (D−P−) and by the size of the D+P+ group. If we assume that the D−P− group represents 50% of a given population, a placebo response rate of 40% (consistent with a 40% rate of D+P+ patients), implies that only 10% of the patients belong to the informative group of D+P− patients, therefore making extraordinarily unlikely the ability to detect any signal. Therefore, it is common for clinical trials to yield uninterpretable results, due in part to the relatively high placebo response, such as in the case

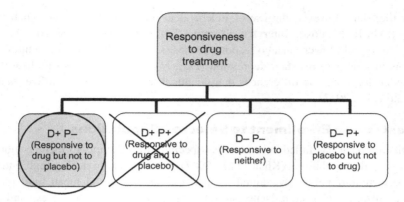

FIGURE 8.1 Subpopulations of patients based on their responsiveness to treatment.

of placebo response rates greater than 40%. In fact, it has been shown that, as symptom reduction with placebo increased, the advantage of the new antidepressant decreased ($r = 0.592$, P < 0.0001) (Khan *et al.*, 2003). It has been suggested that addressing the placebo response issue is one of the most important challenges facing the future of psychopharmacologic drug development.

The placebo response is a major issue in clinical trials for psychiatric disorders. Possible contributing factors to this problem include diagnostic misclassification, issues concerning inclusion/exclusion criteria, outcome measures' lack of sensitivity to change, measurement errors, poor quality of data entry and verification, waxing and waning of the natural course of illness, regression toward the mean phenomenon, patient and clinician expectations about the trial, study design issues, nonspecific therapeutic effects, and high attrition (Fava *et al.*, 2003).

OVERCOMING THE PROBLEM OF EXCESSIVE PLACEBO RESPONSES

Given all the issues outlined above, researchers have been struggling since the 1990s to identify possible remedies for the placebo problem. Specifically, the following approaches have been used to minimize placebo response rates in double-blind clinical trials in psychiatric disorders (Fava *et al.*, 2003).

Standardizing Diagnostic Procedures

Although there is no empirical evidence that improving diagnostic procedures yields lower response rates of placebo, it seems intuitive that the use of structured interviews such as the Structured Clinical Interview for Axis I DSM IV Disorders (SCID) and the Mini-International Neuropsychiatric Interview (MINI) to diagnose psychiatric disorders should help with the issue of diagnostic misclassification. However, even the use of such interviews does not eliminate the possible clinician bias to enroll patients who are not appropriate for the trial. However, the use of independent diagnostic interviews, such as the SAFER diagnostic interview (Targum, Pollack & Fava, 2008), has been shown to yield lower placebo responses rates (less than 20%) in augmentation trials in treatment-resistant depression (Fava *et al.*, 2012) and to significantly greater drug–placebo differences than identical trials that did not utilize them (Ratti *et al.*, 2013).

Restricting Enrollment to Selected Populations

This approach has failed consistently, especially the attempts to include more severely ill populations (Khan *et al.*, 2007). In fact, paradoxically, high entry criteria requirements have failed to increase reliably actual mean total pre-randomization Hamilton Depression Rating Scale (HAM-D) scores, and a greater placebo response was seen in trials requiring higher pre-randomization depressive symptoms (Khan *et al.*, 2007). Therefore, we do not believe that there is any advantage in using this approach, unless the enrichment is based on specific biologic predictors of response to drug treatment, as in the case of pharmacogenetic or brain imaging studies.

Managing Clinicians' Overestimation of Change

In clinical trials, a certain number of enrolled patients may be erroneously included into the trial, and a certain additional number of correctly included patients will be erroneously classified as responders (Schatzberg & Kraemer, 2000). Then, even though there is no actual change in symptoms, these two misidentified groups combine to create an artifactual response rate that is greater than zero (Schatzberg & Kraemer, 2000). There are two general approaches in our field to this issue. One is the management of clinician bias to overestimate severity of symptoms at study entry but not thereafter, and the other one is the management of clinician bias to overestimate improvement at end point. The simplest approach to the first bias is the elimination of severity threshold requirements for inclusion into the trial. Alternatively, researchers have used a variety of tools to address this issue, ranging from the use of self-rating scales to assess severity of illness at entry, to the use of interactive voice response or independent raters (Kobak *et al.*, 1999). Another useful approach is to use outcome measures that can be administered in both clinician- and patient-rated forms, as in the case of the Inventory of Depressive Symptomatology (IDS) (Rush, Carmody & Reimitz, 2000) and the Quick Inventory of Depressive Symptomatology (QIDS) (Uher *et al.*, 2012), therefore allowing concordance between clinician- and self-rated assessments. In such cases, the self-rating measure can be used as the independent validator of the accuracy of the clinician assessment of change.

Rater Training

Since the lower the test–retest reliability of the assessments, the greater this artifactual response rate to placebo can be, rater training programs have proliferated since the 1990s, and such programs have become a standard in the pharmaceutical industry, with very little evidence of their usefulness (Schatzberg & Kraemer, 2000). In fact, a frequent major consequence of this intensive quest for precision and reliability in the use of outcome measures has been the push toward increasingly more detailed and lengthy interviews with patients. It is not uncommon to see didactic videotaped or live interviews where the interviewer takes 35–45 minutes to complete a HAM-D interview. This approach tends to increase the exposure of patients to study clinicians dramatically and can potentially enhance the placebo effect. Although rater training has certainly face validity, one would argue that it is more critical to monitor the accuracy of clinicians' rating, and, therefore, rater monitoring systems have emerged as important tools to complement standard rater training programs.

Requirement of Same Rater

The use of the same rater may be required to increase the reliability of the assessments for each randomized patient from the baseline visit to the endpoint visit. This approach, of course, runs the risk of intensifying the nonspecific therapeutic effects described earlier, in that the continuity of care can only increase the intensity of the therapeutic relationship with the study clinician. It is, therefore, not surprising at all that differences between active comparators and placebo were found to be larger in subjects seen by different raters than in subjects seen by the same rater in depression clinical trials (DeBrota, Gelwicks & Potter, 2002).

Simplification of Study Visits and Assessments

Robinson and Rickels (2000) have recommended shortening the duration of study visits and limiting the number of rating scales to minimize the placebo effect (Robinson & Rickels, 2000). Although intuitively correct, these suggestions have not been tested empirically, but they certainly seem worthy of investigation. In addition, as mentioned earlier, there is a strong possibility of loss of the study's external validity when interactions between clinicians and patients markedly deviate from standard clinical practice. For these reasons, simplification of study visits and assessments appears to be a promising approach to minimizing placebo response.

Minimizing Nonspecific, Therapeutic Effects

Some research groups have attempted to minimize these nonspecific therapeutic effects by preparing scripts to explain the trial to patients and by frequently reminding research staff that 'supportive behaviors' can negatively affect the trials. Whether such approaches help clinical trials remains to be established. As mentioned earlier, it is likely that a secondary effect of a simplification of study visits and assessments is that of a reduction in nonspecific, therapeutic effects.

Placebo Lead-in Phases

Placebo lead-in phases were initially thought to be a useful tool to screen out mood disorder patients who were likely to respond to placebo during the double-blind phase. However, such lead-in phases have been typically single-blinded periods of 1 or 2 weeks, during which the patients are unknowingly treated with placebo, but their clinicians are aware of the placebo treatment. This design may, therefore, potentially lead to clinician biases in underestimating improvement during the lead-in phase, and to verbal/nonverbal communications of low expectation of improvement to patients (e.g., emphasizing strongly to patients that no clinical effect is expected in the first weeks of treatment). It is, therefore, not surprising that the analysis of 75 double-blind trials that had been conducted among patients with major depressive disorder (MDD) and had been published between January 1981 and December 2000, showed no statistically significant association between the proportion of responders to placebo in studies of patients with MDD and the presence of a lead-in phase (Walsh *et al.*, 2002). This is also consistent with the findings by Trivedi and Rush (1994) that the mean placebo response rate of studies that used a placebo lead-in phase did not differ significantly from that of studies that did not use a placebo lead-in.

Extending Trial Duration

After the initial observations by Quitkin (1992) and Quitkin *et al.* (1984) that specific antidepressant drug effects most likely occur after the first 2 weeks of treatment and are stable, while placebo responses tend to occur early and are variable, many researchers have advocated study designs where the duration of the double-blind trial was extended to 8 or 12 weeks for MDD, and for even longer periods for some of the other psychiatric disorders. Whether this approach has led to any reduction in placebo response rates is unclear. Tedeschini, Fava, and Papakostas (2011) pooled the data from 182 drug–placebo comparisons from 104 clinical antidepressant trials (29,213 patients), and found that the strength of the relationship between early and endpoint outcome increased progressively, suggesting the possibility that trials could be shorter. However, only at week 4 did the diagnostic odds ratio (27.44) indicate strong concordance between early and endpoint outcome, suggesting that antidepressant clinical trials cannot be shortened to less than 4 weeks' duration, primarily due to the increased risk of erroneously concluding that an effective treatment is ineffective. Therefore, 4 weeks is the minimum adequate length of a trial in order to reliably detect drug versus placebo differences in MDD. It needs longer time for study continuation therapy, which is used to prevent relapse in MDD. Reimherr *et al.* (1998) reported that patients treated with fluoxetine for 12 weeks whose depressive symptoms remit should continue treatment with fluoxetine for at least an additional 26 weeks to minimize the risk of relapse.

Reducing Number of Sites

Robinson and Rickels (2000) have challenged the current trend favoring very large trials, given that this may be contributing to the escalating placebo response rates plaguing clinical trials today, and have recommended reverting to a simpler development approach, involving a few carefully chosen centers with skilled investigators. This recommendation certainly makes a lot of sense, but it is hard to find quality sites that can also enroll into studies relatively high volume of patients.

Increasing the Sensitivity of Outcome Measures

The greatest experience in this area is probably in MDD trials, where instruments such as the six-item HAM-D, a unidimensional core subscale called the Melancholia scale, has clearly outperformed the gold standard 17-item HAM-D (HAM-D-17) and other longer versions of the HAM-D (O'Sullivan *et al.*, 1997). However, there has been a certain reluctance among trial sponsors to adopt measures that deviate from the current gold standards, and novel scales may be needed.

Reducing the Number of Treatment Arms

A meta-regression (random-effects) of 182 antidepressant trials found that the lesser the probability of receiving placebo (as in the case of studies with two or more active treatments), predicted lesser antidepressant-placebo "efficacy separation" (Papakostas & Fava, 2009). Therefore, since it appears that studies that try simultaneously to evaluate too many potentially active treatments against a placebo may find it more difficult to detect any differences from the placebo, a common approach to clinical trials is now to limit the active treatment arms to one (Schatzberg & Kraemer, 2000).

STANDARD PARALLEL COMPARISON DESIGN

Standard parallel comparison design is a comparative study with an intervention group and a control group and the assignment of the subject to a group is determined by the formal procedure of randomization (Friedman, Furberg & DeMets, 2010) (Figure 8.2).

'Randomization' means randomized allocation of choice of treatment to balance both known and unknown confounders, to ensure comparable risk of outcome at entry to the study. The control may be a standard practice, a placebo, or no intervention at all. It is accepted by medicine as objective scientific methodology that, when ideally performed, produces knowledge untainted by confounding bias (Kaptchuk, 2001).

The basic assumptions of this design are as follows:
1. minimal effects of regression to the mean phenomenon;
2. natural course of illness well-characterized uncommon spontaneous remissions;
3. placebo effect is trivial;
4. expectations about improvement play minor role; and
5. sample's responsiveness to drug is greater than to placebo.

Assumptions of standard parallel comparison designs may not be valid in the studies of mood disorders, because the natural course of the illnesses and placebo effects make a profound influence on study results.

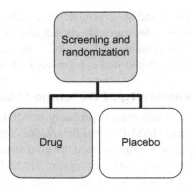

FIGURE 8.2 Standard model design for testing of drugs versus placebo in patients.

Table 8.1 Proportion of Failed Trials of Antidepressants in the Food and Drug Administration (FDA) Data Sets

	Randomized Controlled Trials (#)	Drug > Placebo (%)
New antidepressants	69	31 (45%)
Standard antidepressants	24	14 (58%)
Total	93	45 (48%)

In psychiatry, particularly in antidepressant clinical studies, standard parallel comparison placebo-controlled trials often yield results that are very difficult to interpret because of robust placebo responses. Meta-analyses of trials in MDD suggest that drug–placebo differences in response rates range from 11% to 18% (Yang, Cusin & Fava, 2005). However, in trials of marketed antidepressants present in the US Food and Drug Administration (FDA) databases, antidepressant drugs were superior to placebo in only 45 out of 93 randomized controlled trials (RCTs) (48%), and the placebo response overall appeared to have increased over time (Table 8.1). The frequency of statistically significant differences between antidepressants and placebo was higher in the trials that included patients with more severe depression (Khan *et al.*, 2002). From an extrapolation during the first 6 months of illness, MDD on average, remits in 2% of subjects per week and has spontaneous remission rates of 8–16% over 4–8 weeks (Posternak & Miller, 2001).

SINGLE-BLIND PLACEBO WASHOUT

'Single blind' is a testing procedure in which the administrators do not tell the subjects if they are being given a test treatment or a control treatment in

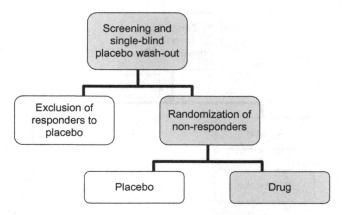

FIGURE 8.3 Single-blind placebo washout followed by randomized parallel comparison.

order to avoid bias in the results. It is commonplace in clinical pharmaceutical research, particularly research involving long-term prophylactic medication, for the period of study of active treatment to be both preceded and followed by a 'washout' period (i.e., a period in which no active treatment is received by the patients entered into a particular trial as subjects) (Figure 8.3).

The specific assumptions of this design are as follows:
1. the clinician's knowledge of the placebo washout does not bias the detection of improvement;
2. the clinician's reduced expectations of change during washout do not get communicated (verbally or not) to the patients;
3. patient's overall expectations of improvement are unaffected.

However, as mentioned earlier, meta-analyses of 101 MDD studies revealed that a placebo run-in does not lower the placebo response rate, increase the drug–placebo difference, and affect the drug response rate postrandomization in either inpatients or outpatients for any antidepressant drug group (Trivedi & Rush, 1994). If there is a postrandomization placebo treatment cell, drug response rates are unchanged or are slightly lower than if there is no placebo treatment cell for outpatients. These results suggest that a pill placebo run-in provides no advantage in acute phase efficacy trials. The single-blind, placebo washout is therefore less effective on clinical trials for mood disorder patients.

CROSSOVER DESIGN

A crossover clinical trial is one in which the effects of different treatments are compared on the same subject during different treatment periods (Hills & Armitage, 1979) (Figure 8.4). Such trials are useful when the treatments are intended to alleviate a condition, rather than affect a cure, so that after the first treatment is withdrawn the subject is in a position to receive a second.

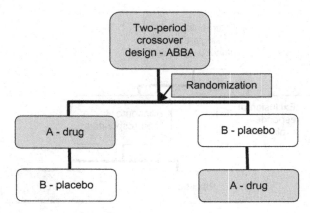

FIGURE 8.4 Two-period crossover design ABBA.

The specific assumptions of this design are as follows:
1. minimal or no carry-over effects;
2. by using subjects as their own controls, statistical power is maximized; and
3. no significant discontinuation reactions.

The main advantages and disadvantages of the crossover design in clinical trials are well known. On the positive side, a comparison of treatments on the same subject is expected to be more precise than a comparison between subjects and, therefore, to require fewer subjects for the same precision. On the negative side, the task of disentangling treatment effects from both time and carry over effects from the previous treatment period can be difficult or even impossible.

ADAPTIVE DESIGNS

Adaptive designs allow planned study modifications based on data accumulating within a study (Kairalla *et al.*, 2012). The promise of greater flexibility and efficiency has clearly generated increasing interest in adaptive designs from clinical, academic, and regulatory parties (Kairalla *et al.*, 2012). The following are adaptive designs that have generated the most current interest.

Randomized Play-the-Winner Clinical Trials

As highlighted in Figure 8.5, this trial design progressively diminishes or eliminates the treatment cells associated with poorer efficacy. The specific assumptions of this design are as follows:
1. the better treatment will actually perform better in the clinical trial;
2. risk of type I error is minimal, and risk can be substantial in some cases;
3. the treatment with better outcome does not cause some serious toxicity; and
4. the degree of placebo response is constant throughout the study.
Of course, the latter assumption is unlikely to be true.

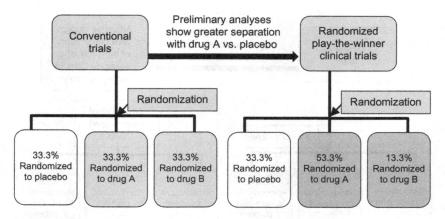

FIGURE 8.5 Randomized play-the-winner clinical trials.

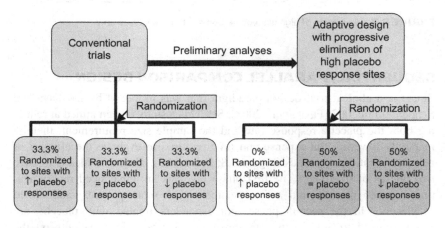

FIGURE 8.6 Progressive elimination of high placebo response sites.

Progressive Elimination of High Placebo Response Sites

As highlighted in Figure 8.6, this trial design progressively diminishes or eliminates the sites associated with higher placebo response rates. The specific assumptions of this design are as follows:

1. the degree of placebo response remains constant at each site; and
2. the clinician's reduced expectations of change do not get communicated (verbally or not) to the patients (e.g., clinicians know that their site would get eliminated based on high placebo responses).

An alternative to this prospective, adaptive design is the use of a retrospective band-pass analysis in multicenter trials (see Figure 8.7), eliminating the sites with placebo responses that are either too high or too low (Merlo-Pich *et al.*, 2010). This approach has shown to enhance the signal detection power in antidepressant trials (Merlo-Pich *et al.*, 2010).

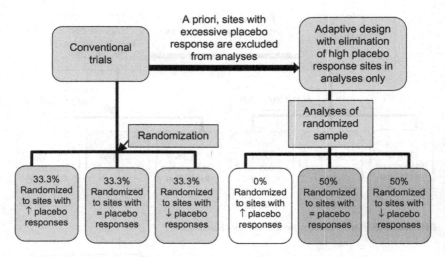

FIGURE 8.7 Elimination of high placebo response sites in analyses only.

SEQUENTIAL, PARALLEL COMPARISON DESIGN

SPCD is a clinical trial design paradigm that was proposed by Dr. Fava and Schoenfeld in 2003 (Fava *et al.*, 2003). SPCD is a study design aimed at reducing both the placebo response rate and the sample size requirement, thereby markedly lowering the expense and time required to evaluate the efficacy of new therapeutic compounds (Figure 8.8; Figure 8.9). The basic idea is to have two phases of treatment. The first phase involves an unbalanced randomization between placebo and active treatment with more patients randomized to placebo. In the second phase, nonresponders treated with placebo are re-randomized to either active treatment or placebo. Since patients on the second phase have already 'failed placebo', their placebo response will be reduced. The analysis pools the data from both phases in order to maximize power and reduce the required sample size.

The first phase is aimed at comparing drug and placebo in a standard parallel comparison design fashion in which drug–placebo differences are expected to be smaller and generating a large cohort of placebo nonresponders. The second phase is aimed at comparing drug and placebo in a parallel comparison design fashion in placebo nonresponders in which drug–placebo differences are expected to be greater, and placebo response is expected to be smaller. The data from the two phases are pooled (including all subjects in phase one and only the placebo nonresponders in phase two) to estimate the drug–placebo differences meaned (in a weighted fashion) across the two phases. When compared with the conventional two-arm clinical trial, SPCD reduces the sample size by at least 50% under a wide range of parameters (Boessen *et al.*, 2012). As shown in Figure 8.10, SPCD trials can also be carried out with pre-randomization to the sequence active–active, placebo–active, and placebo–placebo.

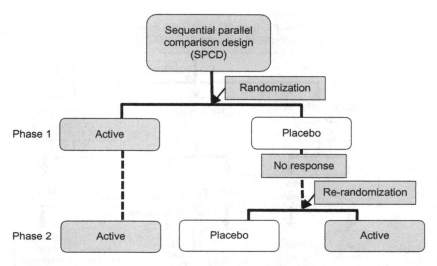

FIGURE 8.8 Sequential, parallel comparison design (SPCD).

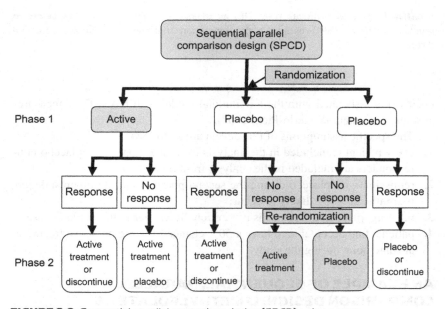

FIGURE 8.9 Sequential, parallel comparison design (SPCD) – three arms.

Each phase can be shortened than standard to increase the feasibility of the trial. There is a marked congruence between end point and half-way drug–placebo differences in standard trials (Yang *et al.*, 2005). According to the meta-analysis by Posternak and Zimmerman (2005), on average, more than 80% of the improvement on placebo occurred in the first half of 6-week trials. The best placebo-responder classification score (86.32% true and 13.68% false

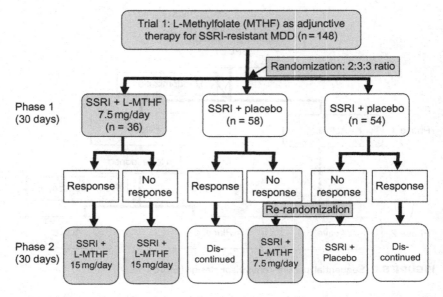

FIGURE 8.10 L-Methylfolate (L-MTHF) as adjunctive therapy for selective serotonin reuptake inhibitor (SSRI)-resistant major depression: trial one. MDD: major depressive disorder.

positive) is associated with the longitudinal model with HAM-D-17 measures at week 4 (Gomeni & Merlo-Pich, 2007).

The specific assumptions of this design are as follows:

1. every patient is included in the analysis from phase one; only placebo non-responders are included in the analysis from phase two;
2. remission with placebo during the second phase in placebo nonresponders is significantly less likely to occur;
3. the drug–placebo difference is proportionally greater in the second phase;
4. patients find acceptable to have a 50% chance of being on active treatment at some point during the study.

AN EXAMPLE OF SEQUENTIAL, PARALLEL COMPARISON DESIGN: L-METHYLFOLATE AS ADJUNCTIVE THERAPY FOR SELECTIVE SEROTONIN REUPTAKE INHIBITOR-RESISTANT MAJOR DEPRESSION

The authors conducted two multicenter SPCD trials to investigate the effect of L-methylfolate (L-MTHF) augmentation in the treatment of MDD in patients who had a partial response or no response to selective serotonin reuptake inhibitors (SSRIs) (Papakostas *et al.*, 2012). In the first trial, 148 outpatients with SSRI-resistant MDD were enrolled in a 60-day study divided into two

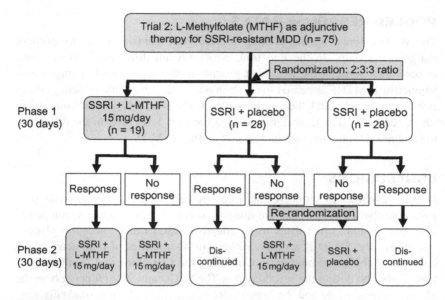

FIGURE 8.11 L-Methylfolate (L-MTHF) as adjunctive therapy for selective serotonin reuptake inhibitor (SSRI)-resistant major depression: trial two. MDD: major depressive disorder.

30-day periods. In the second trial, with 75 patients, the design was identical to the first, except that the L-MTHF dosage was 15 mg/day during both 30-day periods.

Trial One

Eligible patients were randomized to one of three treatment groups in a 2:3:3 ratio. The study was divided into two 30-day phases (phases one and two) (Figure 8.10).

One group of patients (randomization probability 3:8) received two dummy pills identical to L-MTHF in appearance during phases one and two (placebo–placebo group). The second group (randomization probability 3:8) received two dummy pills during phase 1 and one dummy pill and one 7.5-mg L-MTHF pill during phase 2 (placebo–drug group). The third group (randomization probability 2:8) received one dummy pill and one 7.5-mg L-MTHF pill during phase one and two 7.5-mg L-MTHF pills during phase two (drug–drug group). This format of the SPCD was selected instead of the one involving a randomization to drug and placebo in phase one and a re-randomization of placebo nonresponders to drug or placebo in phase two.

Trial Two

The design of the second trial was identical to the first except that the dosing of L-MTHF was 15 mg throughout the trial for all patients receiving it (Figure 8.11).

POOLED RESPONSE RATES

The SPCD model can make pooling of phases one and two on the two primary outcome measures. In the first trial, no significant difference was observed in outcomes between the treatment groups. In the second trial, 15 mg/day of adjunctive L-MTHF appeared to result in a treatment outcome (efficacy) superior to continued SSRI therapy plus placebo in both primary outcome measures, achieving statistical significance at the 0.05 level both in the difference in response rates degree of improvement on the HAM-D.

CONCLUSIONS

Placebo responses in antidepressant trials are very robust. There are many possible contributing factors that are difficult to control. To enhance signal detection, one should enrich trials using adaptive designs and lower the placebo responses. The SPCD is a study design with two phases of treatment, which consist of unbalanced randomization during the first phase and re-randomization of placebo during the second phase. The SPCD aimed at reducing both the placebo response rate and the sample size requirement, thereby markedly lowering the expense and time required to evaluate the efficacy of new therapeutic compounds.

DR. MAURIZIO FAVA'S LIFETIME DISCLOSURES

Research Support:

Abbott Laboratories, Alkermes, Aspect Medical Systems, Astra-Zeneca, BioResearch, BrainCells Inc., Bristol-Myers Squibb Company, Cephalon, Clinical Trial Solutions, LLC, Eli Lilly & Company, EnVivo Pharmaceuticals Inc., Forest Pharmaceuticals Inc., Ganeden, GlaxoSmithKline, J & J Pharmaceuticals, Lichtwer Pharma GmbH, Lorex Pharmaceuticals, NARSAD, NCCAM, NIDA, NIMH, Novartis, Organon Inc., PamLab, LLC, Pfizer Inc, Pharmavite, Roche, Sanofi-Aventis, Shire, Solvay Pharmaceuticals Inc., Synthelabo, and Wyeth-Ayerst Laboratories.

Advisory/Consulting:

Abbott Laboratories, Affectis Pharmaceuticals AG, Amarin, Aspect Medical Systems, Astra-Zeneca, Auspex Pharmaceuticals, Bayer AG, Best Practice Project Management Inc, BioMarin Pharmaceuticals Inc., Biovail Pharmaceuticals Inc., BrainCells Inc, Bristol-Myers Squibb Company, Cephalon, Clinical Trials Solutions, LLC, CNS Response, Compellis, Cypress Pharmaceuticals, Dov Pharmaceuticals, Eisai Inc., Eli Lilly & Company, EPIX Pharmaceuticals, Euthymics Bioscience Inc., Fabre-Kramer Pharmaceuticals Inc., Forest Pharmaceuticals Inc., GlaxoSmithKline, Grunenthal GmBH, Janssen Pharmaceutica, Jazz Pharmaceuticals, J & J Pharmaceuticals, Knoll Pharmaceutical Company, Labopharm, Lorex Pharmaceuticals, Lundbeck, MedAvante Inc., Merck, Methylation Sciences, Neuronetics, Novartis, Nutrition 21, Organon Inc., PamLab, LLC, Pfizer Inc., PharmaStar, Pharmavite,

Precision Human Biolaboratory, Prexa Pharmaceuticals Inc., PsychoGenics, Psylin Neurosciences Inc., Ridge Diagnostics Inc., Roche, Sanofi-Aventis, Sepracor, Schering-Plough, Solvay Pharmaceuticals Inc., Somaxon, Somerset Pharmaceuticals, Synthelabo, Takeda, Tetragenex, TransForm Pharmaceuticals Inc., Transcept Pharmaceuticals, Vanda Pharmaceuticals Inc, Wyeth-Ayerst Laboratories. He has received speaking and publishing honoraria from Adamed, Co., Advanced Meeting Partners, American Psychiatric Association, American Society of Clinical Psychopharmacology, Astra-Zeneca, Belvoir, Boehringer-Ingelheim, Bristol-Myers Squibb Company, Cephalon, Eli Lilly & Company, Forest Pharmaceuticals Inc., GlaxoSmithKline, Imedex, Novartis, Organon Inc., Pfizer Inc, PharmaStar, MGH Psychiatry Academy/ Primedia, MGH Psychiatry Academy/Reed-Elsevier, UBC, and Wyeth-Ayerst Laboratories.

Equity Holdings: Compellis

Royalty/patent, other income: patent applications for SPCD and for a combination of azapirones and bupropionin MDD, copyright royalties for the MGH CPFQ, SFI, ATRQ, DESS, and SAFER

Dr. Hong Jin Jeon's Disclosures:

None

REFERENCES

Boessen, R., Knol, M. J., Groenwold, R. H., et al. (2012). Increasing trial efficiency by early reallocation of placebo nonresponders in sequential parallel comparison designs: Application to antidepressant trials. *Clinical Trials, 9*, 578–587.

DeBrota, D. J., Gelwicks, S. C., Potter, W. Z. (2002). Same rater versus different raters in depression clinical trials. *Proceedings of the 42nd new clinical drug evalution unit annual meeting*, Boca Raton, FL, June 10–13, 2002.

Fava, M., Evins, A. E., Dorer, D. J., et al. (2003). The problem of the placebo response in clinical trials for psychiatric disorders: Culprits, possible remedies, and a novel study design approach. *Psychotherapy and Psychosomatics, 72*, 115–127.

Fava, M., Mischoulon, D., Iosifescu, D., et al. (2012). A double-blind, placebo-controlled study of aripiprazole adjunctive to antidepressant therapy among depressed outpatients with inadequate response to prior antidepressant therapy (ADAPT-A Study). *Psychotherapy and Psychosomatics, 81*, 87–97.

Friedman, L. M., Furberg, C. D., & DeMets, D. L. (2010). *Fundamentals of Clinical Trials* (4th ed.). New York: Springer.

Gomeni, R., & Merlo-Pich, E. (2007). Bayesian modelling and ROC analysis to predict placebo responders using clinical score measured in the initial weeks of treatment in depression trials. *British Journal of Clinical Pharmacology, 63*, 595–613.

Hills, M., & Armitage, P. (1979). The two-period cross-over clinical trial. *British Journal of Clinical Pharmacology, 8*, 7–20.

Kairalla, J. A., Coffey, C. S., Thomann, M. A., et al. (2012). Adaptive trial designs: A review of barriers and opportunities. *Trials, 13*, 145.

Kaptchuk, T. J. (2001). The double-blind, randomized, placebo-controlled trial: Gold standard or golden calf? *Journal of Clinical Epidemiology, 54*, 541–549.

Khan, A., Detke, M., Khan, S. R., et al. (2003). Placebo response and antidepressant clinical trial outcome. *Journal of Nervous and Mental Disease, 191*, 211–218.

Khan, A., Leventhal, R. M., Khan, S. R., et al. (2002). Severity of depression and response to antidepressants and placebo: An analysis of the Food and Drug Administration database. *Journal of Clinical Psychopharmacology, 22*, 40–45.

Khan, A., Schwartz, K., Kolts, R. L., et al. (2007). Relationship between depression severity entry criteria and antidepressant clinical trial outcomes. *Biological Psychiatry, 62,* 65–71.

Kobak, K. A., Greist, J. H., Jefferson, J. W., et al. (1999). Computerized assessment of depression and anxiety over the telephone using interactive voice response. *MD Computing: Computers in Medical Practice, 16,* 64–68.

Merlo-Pich, E., Alexander, R. C., Fava, M., et al. (2010). A new population-enrichment strategy to improve efficiency of placebo-controlled clinical trials of antidepressant drugs. *Clinical Pharmacology and Therapeutics, 88,* 634–642.

O'Sullivan, R. L., Fava, M., Agustin, C., et al. (1997). Sensitivity of the six-item Hamilton Depression Rating Scale. *Acta Psychiatrica Scandinavica, 95,* 379–384.

Papakostas, G. I., & Fava, M. (2009). Does the probability of receiving placebo influence clinical trial outcome? A meta-regression of double-blind, randomized clinical trials in MDD. *European Neuropsychopharmacology, 19,* 34–40.

Papakostas, G. I., Shelton, R. C., Zajecka, J. M., et al. (2012). L-methylfolate as adjunctive therapy for SSRI-resistant major depression: Results of two randomized, double-blind, parallel-sequential trials. *American Journal of Psychiatry, 169,* 1267–1274.

Posternak, M. A., & Miller, I. (2001). Untreated short-term course of major depression: A meta-analysis of outcomes from studies using wait-list control groups. *Journal of Affective Disorders, 66,* 139–146.

Posternak, M. A., & Zimmerman, M. (2005). Is there a delay in the antidepressant effect? A meta-analysis. *Journal of Clinical Psychiatry, 66,* 148–158.

Quitkin, F. M. (1992). Methodology of measuring the efficacy of antidepressants. *Psychopharmacology, 106,* S87–S89.

Quitkin, F. M., Rabkin, J. G., Ross, D., et al. (1984). Identification of true drug response to antidepressants. Use of pattern analysis. *Archives of General Psychiatry, 41,* 782–786.

Ratti, E., Bettica, P., Alexander, R., et al. (2013). Full central neurokinin-1 receptor blockade is required for efficacy in depression: Evidence from orvepitant clinical studies. *Journal of Psychopharmacology, 27,* 424–434.

Reimherr, F. W., Amsterdam, J. D., Quitkin, F. M., et al. (1998). Optimal length of continuation therapy in depression: A prospective assessment during long-term fluoxetine treatment. *American Journal of Psychiatry, 155,* 1247–1253.

Robinson, D. S., & Rickels, K. (2000). Concerns about clinical drug trials. *Journal of Clinical Psychopharmacology, 20,* 593–596.

Rush, A. J., Carmody, T., & Reimitz, P. E. (2000). The Inventory of Depressive Symptomatology (IDS): Clinician (IDS-C) and Self-Report (IDS-SR) ratings of depressive symptoms. *International Journal of Methods in Psychiatric Research, 9,* 49–59.

Schatzberg, A. F., & Kraemer, H. C. (2000). Use of placebo control groups in evaluating efficacy of treatment of unipolar major depression. *Biological Psychiatry, 47,* 736–744.

Targum, S. D., Pollack, M. H., & Fava, M. (2008). Redefining affective disorders: Relevance for drug development. *CNS Neuroscience & Therapeutics, 14,* 2–9.

Tedeschini, E., Fava, M., & Papakostas, G. I. (2011). Placebo-controlled, antidepressant clinical trials cannot be shortened to less than 4 weeks' duration: A pooled analysis of randomized clinical trials employing a diagnostic odds ratio-based approach. *Journal of Clinical Psychiatry, 72,* 98–113.

Trivedi, M. H., & Rush, H. (1994). Does a placebo run-in or a placebo treatment cell affect the efficacy of antidepressant medications? *Neuropsychopharmacology, 11,* 33–43.

Uher, R., Perlis, R. H., Placentino, A., et al. (2012). Self-report and clinician-rated measures of depression severity: Can one replace the other? *Depression and Anxiety, 29,* 1043–1049.

Walsh, B. T., Seidman, S. N., Sysko, R., et al. (2002). Placebo response in studies of major depression: Variable, substantial, and growing. *JAMA, 287,* 1840–1847.

Yang, H., Cusin, C., & Fava, M. (2005). Is there a placebo problem in antidepressant trials? *Current Topics in Medicinal Chemistry, 5,* 1077–1086.

Chapter | Nine

Rating Scales in Bipolar Disorder

Martha Sajatovic,[1] Peijun Chen[1,2] and Robert C. Young[3]

[1]*Case Western Reserve University School of Medicine, Cleveland, OH, USA;*
[2]*Louis Stokes Cleveland VA Medical Center, Cleveland, OH, USA;*
[3]*Weill Cornell Medical College, New York, NY, USA*

CHAPTER OUTLINE

Clinical Trial Design Challenges in Mood Disorders. DOI: http://dx.doi.org/10.1016/B978-0-12-405170-6.00009-9

INTRODUCTION

Over their lifespan, individuals with bipolar disorder (BD) typically experience a constellation of problems and symptoms related to their mood disorder, comorbid conditions, and burdens or challenges related to BD. It is this highly variable presentation that complicates assessment, delays definitive diagnosis in many cases, and makes determination of outcomes particularly challenging. There are several standardized measures that are used to evaluate clinical status in people with BD, and application of these measures, particularly when applied longitudinally, can help to evaluate status or outcomes in patients who have a condition that is inherently dynamic. Manic or hypomanic symptoms are a necessary occurrence for bipolar diagnosis, while depressive symptoms appear to be pervasive and cause an inordinate disability and heavily impact quality of life (Judd *et al.*, 2005). In addition to manic and depressive symptoms, individuals with BD can have concurrent anxiety symptoms, sleep problems, and use of legal or illicit substance that may be an additional focus of treatment (IRBD, 2012).

Evaluation of effectiveness of treatments in BD commonly focuses on change in manic or depressive symptoms and the majority of standardized BD assessments focus on mood symptoms severity (Picardi, 2009; Sajatovic & Ramirez, 2013). Other important dimensions of status and outcome that can be assessed with standardized ratings include screening for BD, categorization of response to treatment, quality of life, somatic symptoms that may be related to biologic therapies, and evaluations used broadly in psychiatric populations such as global psychopathology. Knowledge of available standardized rating scales for the assessment of patients with BD can help clinicians and researchers to choose the most appropriate instruments for their specific needs.

This chapter will discuss standardized rating scales that are specific to BD or general scales that are commonly used in the assessment of patients with BD. We will review published reports of standardized rating in bipolar mania and depression as well as clinical criteria that are based upon the use of standardized rating scales. The chapter includes a focus on selected instruments originally developed for use in populations with diagnoses other than BD that are commonly used in bipolar research studies, as well as use of rating scales in individuals with BD across the lifespan. Finally, the chapter will conclude with a summary of anticipated future directions in applications of rating scales in bipolar clinical trials and recommendations for future research.

SCREENING INSTRUMENTS FOR BIPOLAR DISORDER

Building on earlier work, investigators since the 1990s have devised tools that may be used to screen for BD in psychiatric patient populations. These have emphasized self-report, and are envisioned as a cost-effective strategy. It is important to remember that screening instruments are intended to identify individuals who may have a given disorder and that they should always be followed by a careful clinical assessment in order to derive a definitive diagnosis.

General Behavioral Inventory

Depue *et al.* (1989) modified a self-inventory, originally developed for identification of adolescents and young adults at risk for BD, to identify unipolar and bipolar affective conditions. The General Behavioral Inventory (GBI) instrument has 46 unipolar items and 26 bipolar items.

With respect to selected psychometric properties, in a university sample, the unipolar and bipolar scales of this version of the GBI were found to have adequate sensitivity (0.78 and 0.76, respectively) and specificity (0.99 and 0.99, respectively).

Manic Depressiveness Scale

Thalbourne, Delin and Bassett (1994) and Thalbourne and Bassett (1998) initially presented this self-report instrument as a 19-item questionnaire regarding history of manic and depressive experiences. It was later converted to an 18-item instrument with equivalent number of items for each mood state. Reliability and consistency of the original scale were adequate. Distributions of scores overlapped between bipolar patients and controls, however. Scores for the modified scale were significantly correlated with number of hospitalizations and severity for bipolar patients but not unipolar depressed patients.

Mood Disorder Questionnaire

Based on Diagnostic and Statistical Manual of Mental Disorders, Fourth Edition (DSM-IV) criteria (American Psychiatric Association, 2000), the self-report Mood Disorder Questionnaire (MDQ) has 13 yes–no items, and two questions verifying clustering of symptoms and that the episodes caused problems (Hirschfeld, 2002). Experience with ambulatory psychiatric patients with Structured Clinical Interview for DSM IV Disorders (SCID)-verified BD found a sensitivity of 0.73 and a specificity of 0.90. However, a population-based replication study found a much lower sensitivity. In community or primary care settings, the MDQ may rule out BD but may not rule it in.

Bipolar Affective Disorder Dimensional Scale

The Bipolar Affective Disorder Dimensional Scale (BADDS) is a numerical rating system that was designed to be an adjunct to categorical best estimate lifetime diagnosis procedures (Craddock *et al.*, 2004). Four dimensions are each rated on a 0 to 100 scale. These are mania, depression, psychosis, and incongruence. Criteria are presented for ranges of scores within each dimension. The scale is completed by experienced clinicians. The authors calculated intraclass correlations using 20 case vignettes reviewed by nine raters: mean agreements with consensus ratings were 0.96, 0.90, 0.86, and 0.89 in the four dimensions. When a separate group of seven clinicians reviewed vignettes of 20 diagnostically challenging cases, the Cohen's kappa was 0.68 and 0.62 for DSM-IV and International Classification of Diseases (ICD)-10 categorical agreement, respectively; mean agreements on the BADDS dimensions were 0.91, 0.86, 0.96, and 0.78.

Bipolar Spectrum Diagnostic Scale

The Bipolar Spectrum Diagnostic Scale (BSDS) scale consists of a descriptive story that contains features of bipolar illness, and to which the patient may assent on a sentence by sentence basis (Ghaemi *et al.*, 2005). In patients with BD or unipolar major depression, the sensitivity for BD was 0.76 and the specificity was 0.85. A shift in threshold was associated with an increased specificity to 0.93 without significant loss of sensitivity.

Screening Assessment of Depression-Polarity

The Screening Assessment of Depression-Polarity (SAD-P) is a three-item instrument, developed to screen for BD in patients suffering from acute major depression (Solomon *et al.*, 2006). It assesses presence of delusions during the current episode, number of prior episodes of major depression, and family history of major depression or mania. Sensitivities of 0.72–0.82 for bipolar depression were found in a cross-validated sample of patients with unipolar or bipolar illness.

MANIA SCALES

Review of Instruments

The advent of pharmacologic and other somatic treatments for BD stimulated attention on the need for assessment instruments, in particular for manic states. These states are a hallmark of BD and were seen as a target for lithium treatment in particular. Mania scales were seen as a necessary advance over nonspecific instruments such as the Brief Psychiatric Rating Scale (BPRS) (Overall & Gorham, 1962), which was found to be insensitive to manic psychopathology (Shopsin *et al.*, 1975). Most literature involves the use of observer/interview-based instruments.

Description of Specific Instruments

RATER-ADMINISTERED MANIA SCALES

Manic State Rating Scale

The Manic State Rating Scale (MSRS) was developed at the National Institute of Mental Health (NIMH) (Beigel, Murphy & Bunney, 1971; Murphy *et al.*,

1974). It is a 26-item instrument intended to be completed by trained nurse observers. Each item is rated from 0 to 5 on both frequency and intensity. The numbers of items and nurse training have been considered limiting factors for applications outside of a research unit.

Selected psychometric properties: the authors reported high inter-rater reliability (0.84–0.99). They also reported high concurrent validity when total scores were compared with a 15-item scale rated by psychiatrists, and a 14-item scale completed by nurses.

Time to complete: 15–30 minutes.

Modified Manic Rating Scale

The Modified Manic Rating Scale (MMRS) is a 28-item scale intended for use based on interview and other information (Blackburn, Loudon & Ashworth, 1977; Loudon, Blackburn & Ashworth, 1977). The items were based primarily on the MSRS. The item scoring is based on anchor points.

Selected psychometric properties: inter-rater reliability was demonstrated among three raters in 16 patients ($r = 0.79$–0.85). All individual item scores were significantly correlated with total score except for the 'is depressed' item (0.24). Validity was supported by significant correlations between MMRS total and global ratings by nurses (0.65) and by physicians (0.80).

Time to complete: 30–45 minutes.

Petterson Scale

The authors of the Petterson Scale (PS) created a brief instrument that consists of seven items, each with five grades of severity based on clinical descriptions (Petterson, Fyro & Sedvall, 1973). One limitation of the PS is that assessment of sleep disturbance is not included.

Selected psychometric properties: inter-rater reliability pretreatment was 0.80 for the total score and ranged from 0.57 to 1.0. The total scores and all item scores decreased rapidly and significantly with treatment.

Time to complete: 15–30 minutes.

Young Mania Rating Scale

The Young Mania Rating Scale (YMRS) is an 11-item interviewer rated scale (Young et al., 1978). Ratings can include other sources of information. The items have five defined grades of severity. Four items are double weighted (irritability, speech, thought content and disruptive/aggressive behavior). The scale was modeled on the Hamilton Rating Scale for Depression (HAM-D). The YMRS is by far the most commonly used standardized measure of bipolar manic symptoms in acute mania clinical trials.

Selected psychometric properties: the scale is intended for use by clinically experienced raters. Inter-rater reliability reported by the authors was adequate for total score (0.93) and for individual items ranged from 0.67 to 0.95. They presented validation using concurrent global ratings and ratings with other mania rating scales.

Time to complete: about 15 minutes.

Bech-Rafaelsen Scale

The Bech-Rafaelsen Scale (BRMS) is an 11-item scale. Each item has five-points of specified severity (Bech, 2002; Bech *et al.*, 1979).

Selected psychometric properties: the authors reported good inter-rater reliability: comparison of total scores of each rater with the mean scores of other raters yielded a rho of 0.97–0.99. They also demonstrated high item homogeneity by comparisons with total score ($r = 0.72$–0.94 for all items except sleep, which was 0.48).

Time to complete: 15–30 minutes.

Mania Rating Scale

The Mania Rating Scale (MRS) (Endicott & Spitzer, 1978) is an 11-item instrument derived from the Change Scale embedded within the widely used Schedule for Affective Disorders and Schizophrenia (SADS).

Selected psychometric properties: those investigators report high ($r > 0.90$) inter-rater and test–retest reliability on the manic syndrome summary scale. Internal consistency (Cronbach's alpha) was similarly high.

Time to complete: 15 minutes.

Mania Diagnostic and Severity Scale

The Mania Diagnostic and Severity Scale (MADS) was developed as part of the National Institutes of Health (NIH) Biological Collaborative studies of the neurobiology of mood disorders (Secunda *et al.*, 1985). It was constructed from items contained in the SADS-C (Spitzer & Endicott, 1978), and items selected from both the Video Interview Behavior Evaluation Scale (VIBES) (Katz & Itil, 1974) and a nursing observation instrument, the Affective Disorders Rating Scale (ADRS) (Murphy *et al.*, 1982). The investigators presented the 23 items of the MADS, together with a set of related categorical outcome criteria. The nature of this instrument limits application in many clinical contexts.

Selected psychometric properties: Secunda *et al.* (1985) also presented satisfactory mean intraclass correlations for three of the components of the MADS: 0.89 for the VIBES-B2 items, and 0.85 and 0.91 for the ADRS-1 and ADRS-2 items, respectively. They also presented evidence for discriminant validity and for sensitivity to change during treatment.

Time to complete: more than 60 minutes.

Clinician Administered Rating Scale for Mania

The authors developed the 15-item Clinician Administered Rating Scale for Mania (CARS-M), each item scored on a 0–5 continuum (Altman *et al.*, 1994). In addition to information guiding selection of grades of severity, an overall instruction regarding each item is provided. Separate items for delusions and hallucinations are included.

Selected psychometric properties: the authors obtained evidence of good inter-rater reliability for five raters viewing 14 videotaped interviews; the intraclass correlations for the item scores ranged from 0.54 to 0.99 with a mean of 0.81. They also demonstrated test–retest reliability, performed a factor analysis, and demonstrated discriminant validity against other diagnostic groups.

Time to complete: 15–30 minutes.

Clinical Global Impression-Bipolar

The Clinical Global Impression-Bipolar (CGI-BP) instrument (Spearing *et al.*, 1997) was developed as an extension of the Clinical Global Impression (CGI) (Guy, 1976) for BD, with the intent to include better guidance in scoring. It has three scales: mania, depression, and an overall scale. Each is rated separately on cross-sectional global severity, change from baseline, and change from worst phase of current episode. The conceptual advantage of a global scoring system is to permit consideration of all aspects of mental status and behavior considered relevant by the clinician rater. To address the risk of low inter-rater agreement the authors provided users' guides.

Selected psychometric properties: 11 clinicians trained in the use of the CGI-BP rated videotapes of five patients. Intraclass correlation for mania, depression, and overall cross-sectional severity were 1.0, 0.92, and 0.93, respectively.

Time to complete: less than 5 minutes after a clinical assessment.

PATIENT-RATED MANIA SCALES

Self-report instruments applied to manic states have generated a more limited literature than observer/clinician-rated scales. In moderate to severely ill patients, factors such as poor cooperation, inattention, and lack of insight can limit their application. Self-report mania scales have generally not been included in clinical trials.

Visual Analog Scales

The visual analog scales method for reporting internal state has a long history (Hayes & Patterson, 1921; Zealley & Aitken, 1969). The symptom being evaluated is generally assessed by placing a mark on a 100-mm line having opposite descriptors at either end. Advantages include rapidity of completion and low participant burden. Ahearn and Carroll (1996) presented a 23-item assessment tool called the Multiple Visual Analogue Scales for Bipolarity (MVAS). Bauer *et al.* (2000) applied the visual analog scale format in a revised 15-item Internal State Scale (ISS).

Selected psychometric properties: Ahearn and Carroll (1996) found that test–retest reliability was adequate for MVAS, although correlation coefficients were higher for total scores in unipolar (mean 0.85) than in bipolar patients (mean 0.70). Bauer *et al.* (2000) reported moderate agreement (kappa = 0.55–0.56) between ISS and clinician classifications of mood states, using alternative ISS classification criteria.

Time to complete: 10 minutes.

M-D Scale

The M-D Scale (M-DS) is an early instrument designed to assess features of BD. This scale requires a yes/no response to a series of statements (Plutchik *et al.*, 1970). Sixteen out of an original 50 items were found to differentiate manic or hypomanic mood states from euthymic states in a series of patients tested longitudinally.

Selected psychometric properties: there was internal consistency in responses on the mania subscale, assessed by a split half comparison ($r = 0.83$).

Time to complete: 5 minutes.

Self-Report Mania Inventory

The Self-Report Mania Inventory (SRMI) is a 47-item instrument consisting of statements answered true or false (Shugar *et al.*, 1992).

Selected psychometric properties: scores on the scale differentiated manic patients from patients with other diagnoses. Responses on the items showed internal consistency. Factor analysis generated two factors. Test–retest reliability was high (0.93).

Time to complete: 15 minutes.

Affective Self-Rating Scale

The Affective Self-Rating Scale (ASRS) scale has nine mania items and nine depressed items. Each item is rated from 0 to 4 (Adler *et al.*, 2008).

Selected psychometric properties: internal consistency in the mania subscale was high, as indicated by Cronbach's alpha of 0.91.

Time to complete: 5 minutes.

Altman Self-Report Mania Rating Scale

The Altman Self-Report Mania Rating Scale (ASRM) consists of 13 items each consisting of five statements ordered from 0 to 4. The statements describe increasingly manic symptoms/behaviors (Altman, Hedeker, Peterson & Davis, 1997).

Selected psychometric properties: three factors were derived. The test–retest reliability was high ($r = 0.86$–0.89) for all three of these subscales. Concurrent validity was supported by correlations with interview-based scales (CARS-M and YMRS). Scores on the mania subscale were higher in bipolar mania than in comparison groups with other diagnoses.

Time to complete: 5 minutes.

MANIA SCALES IN CLINICAL TRIALS AND RELATED LITERATURE

Table 9.1 gives examples of clinical trial publications in which various mania scales were used as outcome measures. Relatively few of the scales listed above were used in such trials. The table also indicates the frequency of publications in which the scales have cited in the general literature to give an approximate idea of scale recognition.

Table 9.1 Observer/Interviewer-Rated Scales for Mania

Scale	Key Features	Representative Clinical Trial/Study	Citations
BRMS	11 items: motor activity, verbal activity, flight of thoughts, voice/noise level, hostility/destructiveness, mood (feelings of wellbeing), self-esteem, contact with others, sleep changes, sexual interest, and work activities Clinician rated	Grunze *et al.*, 1999	244
CARS-M	15 items: elevated mood, irritability/aggressiveness, hypermotor activity, pressured speech, flight of ideas/racing thoughts, distractibility, grandiosity, decreased need for sleep, excessive energy, poor judgment, disordered thinking, delusions, hallucinations, orientation, insight Clinician rated	Janicak *et al.*, 2001	92
CGI-BP	3 domains: mania, depression, overall Each with 3 items	Berwaerts *et al.*, 2012	417
MADS	23 items Sources: Clinical interview ratings, videotape ratings, nurse ratings	Swann *et al.*, 1986	110
MMRS	28 items Clinician rated	Shafti, 2010	72
MRS	Derived from SADS Change Scale 11 items: elevated mood, reduced need for sleep, more energetic, increased activity, motor hyperactivity, pressured speech, racing thoughts, grandiosity, overt anger, poor judgment, lack of insight Clinician rated	Bowden *et al.*, 1994	37
MSRS	26 items Rated by trained nurses	Lerer *et al.*, 1987	132
PS	7 items: motor activity, pressure of speech, noisiness, flight of ideas, aggressiveness, orientation, elevated mood Clinician rated	Garza-Trevino, Overall & Hollister, 1992	69
YMRS	11 items: elevated mood, activity-energy, sleep, sexual interest, speech, irritability, language-thought disorder, abnormal mental content, disruptive-aggressive behavior, appearance, insight Clinician rated	Hirschfeld *et al.*, 1999	2470

Numbers of citations were obtained using Web of Knowledge (Thompson Reuters): All three citation databases: Science Citation Index – Expanded (1900–present); Social Sciences Citation Index (1956–present); Arts and Humanities Citation Index (1975–present). Citations were only English language publications.
BRMS: Bech-Rafaelsen Scale; CARS-M: Clinician Administered Rating Scale for Mania; CGI-BP: Clinical Global Impression-Bipolar Disorder; MADS: Mania Diagnostic and Severity Scale; MMRS: Modified Manic Rating Scale; MRS: Mania Rating Scale; MSRS: Manic State Rating Scale; PS: Petterson Scale; SADS: Schedule for Affective Disorders and Schizophrenia; YMRS: Young Mania Rating Scale.

DEPRESSION SCALES IN BIPOLAR DISORDER

Review of Instruments

Judd and colleagues (2002) reported that patients with BD experience depressive symptoms more than three times longer than they experience bipolar manic symptoms. Yet in spite of the pervasiveness of bipolar depressive symptoms, there are fewer bipolar depression clinical trials than mania trials (Fountoulakis *et al.*, 2012), and there is a paucity of measures specifically developed for the assessment of depressive symptoms in individuals with BD. The Schedule for Affective Disorders and Schizophrenia (SADS), a structured diagnostic instrument focused on DSM criteria, has a version that includes a 'change' item (SADS-C) (Spitzer & Endicott, 1978), which evaluates symptom severity change over the past 7 days. However, a potential barrier to wider application of the SADS in clinical trials is the need for fairly intensive training prior to implementation, and use of the SADS-C to assess bipolar depressive symptoms in clinical trials is limited (Freeman *et al.*, 1992).

The most commonly used instruments in contemporary bipolar depression clinical trials are the HAM-D (Hamilton, 1960) and the Montgomery Äsberg Depression Rating Scale (MADRS) (Berk *et al.*, 2004; Calabrese *et al.*, 2008; Montgomery & Äsberg, 1979; Weisler *et al.*, 2008). Both the HAM-D and MADRS were developed in the 1960s and 1970s and were intended for use in patients with unipolar depression.

Several bipolar depression clinical trials use both the HAM-D and the MADRS (Calabrese *et al.*, 1999, 2008). As noted by Berk and colleagues (2007), while the HAM-D and MADRS are often considered 'gold' or 'global' standards for measurement of depressive severity and correlate well with instruments that are used to measure general psychopathology in depression clinical trials (Dorz *et al.*, 2003; Guy, 1976), these instruments have a number of problematic elements for bipolar clinical trials given that they were not developed or originally intended for assessment of bipolarity. Neither the MADRS nor the HAM-D specifically evaluates manic or hypomanic that can occur in individuals with bipolar depression. Illustrative of the common occurrence of concomitant depressive and manic/hypomanic symptoms, a treatment trial involving individuals with type I bipolar depression found rates of mixed symptoms in the order of 45–49% with the most frequent mixed symptoms in bipolar depression being irritability, reduced need for sleep, talkativeness, and racing thoughts (Benazzi *et al.*, 2009). Given the limitations of the HAM-D and the MADRS in assessing mixed symptoms, a typical strategy in bipolar depression clinical trials is to add a mania scale such as the YMRS to capture both baseline mixed symptoms as well as emergent manic or hypomanic symptoms.

In addition to their lack of specificity for bipolar depression, the MADRS and HAM-D do not assess the full spectrum of symptoms that may be particularly common in bipolar individuals such as hyperphagia or hypersomnia (Berk *et al.*, 2004). Other clinically relevant symptoms that accompany BD may also be missed or under-detected. It is increasingly evident that cognitive impairments can be seen even in the euthymic phase of BD. While there are conflicting data, a review by Robinson and Ferrier (2006) suggests that there may be a significant negative relationship between cumulative number of bipolar depressive episodes and various measures of neuropsychologic function.

More recently, and in response to limitations in existing instruments, a depression assessment specific to BD has been developed by Berk and colleagues that is attentive to the phenomenological nuances of bipolar depression (Berk *et al.*, 2004, 2007; Galvao *et al.*, 2013), the Bipolar Depression Rating Scale (BDRS). While promising, the BDRS has not been widely used in bipolar depression clinical trials (Berk *et al.*, 2008).

Description of Specific Instruments for Measuring Depressive Symptoms in Bipolar Disorder

RATER-ADMINISTERED DEPRESSION SCALES USED IN BIPOLAR STUDIES

Hamilton Rating Scale for Depression

The HAM-D is an observer-rated scale that evaluates core symptoms of depression (Bagby *et al.*, 2004; Hamilton, 1960, 1967, 1976; Snaith, 1996). While there are multiple versions of the HAM-D, versions consisting of 17–21 items (including two, two-part items, weight and diurnal variation) are most common in clinical trials. A grid version of the HAM-D that uses structure interview prompts and standardized scoring has been developed to advance implementation of HAM-D assessment in clinical trials (Bagby *et al.*, 2004; Kalai *et al.*, 2002). Scoring for all versions of the HAM-D is based upon the clinical interview, plus any additional available information such as reports from significant others or family. Scoring ranges on a 0 to 4 spectrum (0 = none/absent and 4 = most severe) or a 0 to 2 spectrum (0 = absent/none and 2 = severe). A modified version of the scale with anchor points is contained in the ECDEU manual published by the U.S. National Institute of Mental Health (Guy, 1976). The HAM-D heavily weights consideration of somatic symptoms of depression such as sleep and appetite and could be substantially (and perhaps inappropriately) affected by medical comorbidity that is commonly seen among individuals with BD. The total score on the HAM-D in bipolar clinical trials generally consists of only the sum of the first 17 items. A global consensus statement on recommendations for standards in bipolar depression research studies suggests that the minimum score for entry into a bipolar depression trial should be operationalized as a score of greater than 20 on the 17-item HAM-D, while efficacy is best tested in individuals who have baseline total HAM-D scores of greater than 24 (Goodwin *et al.*, 2008). Strengths of the HAM-D include its excellent validation/research base, and ease of administration. The HAM-D has been translated into nearly all European languages, and is readily used in international clinical trials.

Selected psychometric properties: internal consistency of the HAM-D is reported to be 0.76–0.92. Inter-rater reliability on HAM-D total scores range from 0.87 to 0.95. This may be improved upon with two experienced raters working together. A concern with validity in BD is that some clinical features such as somatic symptoms may not be mood-related and could contribute to total scores being a misleading index of bipolar depression severity.

Time to complete scale: 20–30 minutes.

Montgomery Äsberg Depression Rating Scale

The MADRS, drawn from the Comprehensive Psychopathological Rating Scale (CPRS) (Äsberg et al., 1978), consists of 10 items evaluating core symptoms of depression (Montgomery & Äsberg, 1979; Montgomery et al., 1978). Nine of the items are based upon patient report, and one is on the rater's observation during the rating interview. MADRS items are rated on a 0–6 continuum (0 = no abnormality, 6 = severe). The MADRS is relatively quick to administer, and unlike the HAM-D, does not focus predominately on the somatic symptoms of depression, but rather addresses core mood symptoms such as sadness, tension, lassitude, pessimistic thoughts, and suicidal thoughts. A limitation of the MADRS in bipolar clinical trials is its absence of focus on common bipolar depressive symptoms such as feelings of worthlessness, anhedonia, and motor retardation (Berk et al., 2004).

Selected psychometric properties: there appears to be relatively good correlation between MADRS and HAM-D scores. Inter-rater reliability on the MADRS with different pairs of raters has been reported to be 0.89–0.97. Inter-rater reliability between raters of different disciplines (psychiatrist/nurse) has also been demonstrated to be good.

Time to complete scale: 15–20 minutes.

Inventory of Depressive Symptomatology

The Inventory of Depressive Symptomatology (IDS) is a standardized, 30-item, rater-administered scale to evaluate depressive severity using DSM-IV criteria (Rush et al., 1996; Trivedi et al., 2004). The IDS is available in 28- and 30-item versions with formats that have been developed for self-rating (IDS-SR) and rating by clinicians (IDS-C). The 30-item version of the IDS-C30 includes items in the 28-item version plus the addition of items for interpersonal sensitivity and leaden paralysis/lack of physical energy. The IDS-C30 is intended to reference the last 7 days prior to administration of the scale. Responses are scored on a 4-point continuum (0 = no abnormality, 4 = greatest severity) with well-defined anchor points. A semistructured interview guide provides prompts to assist in comprehensively assessing each item. Training videos in the use of the IDS are available from the scale developer and the scale has been translated into multiple languages including French, German, Spanish, Romanian, and Japanese.

Selected psychometric properties: the IDS were validated on a wide range of patients including individuals with dysthymic disorder. Cronbach's alpha is reported as 0.94 for the IDS-C30 based upon assessment of large groups of symptomatic and remitted patients. Internal consistency was lower only among

symptomatic patients (0.67 for the IDS-C30). The IDS-C30 is highly correlated with the HAM-D and Beck Depression Inventory (BDI).
Time to complete scale: 30 minutes.

Bipolar Depression Rating Scale

The BDRS is a 20-item instrument specifically developed for the assessment
of bipolar depressive symptoms (Berk *et al.*, 2004, 2007; Cahill *et al.*, 2005).
A strength of the BDRS is its ability to assess mixed symptoms and atypical
symptoms of depression. The developers have established validity in modestly
sized samples of adults with DSM-IV BD who were all in a current depressive
episode. The scale was developed to be administered by psychiatrists or other
trained raters. Symptom severity is operationalized along a 4-item continuum
(0 = no symptoms present, 1 = mild, 2 = moderate, 3 = severe). A detailed
semistructured scoring manual has been developed that provides operationalized anchor points. Both the BDRS itself and the scoring manual are available from the scale developer at: http://www.barwonhealth.org.au/research/
column-3/bipolar-depression-rating-scale-bdrs (last accessed 31 July 2014).
While promising, the BDRS still needs to be tested more broadly in clinical
trials.

Selected psychometric properties: the BDRS has very good internal consistency with a reported Cronbach's alpha of 0.917 and strong correlations coefficients with the MADRS ($r = 0.906$) and HAM-D ($r = -0.744$) and the mixed
subscale correlated with the YMRS ($r = 0.757$). The BDRS appears to have
good internal validity and adequate inter-rater reliability can be achieved.
Time to complete scale: 15 minutes.

PATIENT-RATED DEPRESSION SCALES USED IN BIPOLAR STUDIES
Quick Inventory of Depressive Symptomatology

The Quick Inventory of Depressive Symptomatology (QIDS) (Merikangas
et al., 2007; Rush *et al.*, 2003) was originally developed as a 16-item self-rated
depression assessment battery derived from the larger, 30-item rater-administered IDS (Rush *et al.*, 1996). The QIDS includes items associated with the
nine symptom domains used to define a major depressive episode as per the
DSM-IV. The scale is available in clinician (QIDS-C 16) and self-rated versions (QIDS-SR 16) and is based on the 7-day period prior to the time of scale
administration. Total scores range from 0 to 27 and are the sum of scores for
each of nine symptom domains, which are depressed mood, loss of interest
or pleasure, concentration/decision making, self-outlook, suicidal ideation,
energy/fatigability, sleep, weight/appetite change, and psychomotor changes.
Higher scores indicate more severe depressive severity.

In a study by Merikangas and colleagues (2007), bipolar depression symptom severity was assessed using the QIDS-SR (Rush *et al.*, 2003). Standard
QIDS-SR cutoff points were used to define mood episodes as severe (including original QIDS-SR ratings of very severe, with ratings in the range 16 and

greater on the QIDS-SR), moderate (11–15 on the QIDS-SR), mild (6–10 on the QIDS-SR), or not clinically significant (0–5 on the QIDS-SR). As with the rater-administered MADRS and HAM-D, limitations of the QIDS include the lack of focus on mixed symptoms and lack of specificity for atypical depressive symptoms that may be particularly common in individuals with BD.

Selected psychometric properties: in one study comparing the psychometric properties of the QIDS-SR and the 24-item HAM-D in adults with major depression, internal consistency was high for the QIDS-SR (Rush *et al.*, 2003) (Cronbach's alpha = 0.86) and the HAM-D (Cronbach's alpha = 0.88). QIDS-SR total scores were highly correlated with HAM-D (0.86) total scores. About 1.3 times the QIDS-SR total score is predictive of the 17-item version of the HAM-D total score. The QIDS-SR also appears to be sensitive to symptom change (Rush *et al.*, 2003).

Time to complete scale: 5–10 minutes.

Beck Depression Inventory

The Beck Depression Inventory (BDI) is a 21-item, self-rated scale that evaluates key symptoms of depression including mood, pessimism, sense of failure, self-dissatisfaction, guilt, punishment, self-dislike, self-accusation, suicidal ideas, crying, irritability, social withdrawal, indecisiveness, body image change, work difficulty, insomnia, fatigability, loss of appetite, weight loss, somatic preoccupation, and loss of libido (Beck & Steer, 1993; Beck, Steer & Garbing, 1988). Individual scale items are scored on a 4-point continuum (0 = least, 3 = most), with a total summed score range of 0–63. Higher scores indicate greater depressive severity. Two subscales include a cognitive-affective subscale and a somatic-performance subscale.

Selected psychometric properties: mean internal-consistency estimates of the total scores are 0.86 for psychiatric patients. The BDI mean correlation of total score with clinical ratings of depression is greater than 0.60. In bipolar depression trials, the BDI would generally be a secondary outcome measure typically paired with a commonly used rater-administered scale such as the HAM-D (Saricicek *et al.*, 2011).

Time to complete scale: 5–10 minutes.

Depression Scales in Clinical Trials and Related Literature

Table 9.2 illustrates the use of selected common measures used in clinical trials to assess bipolar depression.

OTHER RELEVANT DIMENSIONS OF BIPOLAR OUTCOME IN CLINICAL TRIALS

There has been a rapid increase in the number of bipolar clinical trials in the 2000s. Based on the results of these studies, approximately a dozen psychotropic

Table 9.2 Rating Scales for Depression in Bipolar Disorder

Scale	Type	Key Features	Representative Clinical Trials	Citation Index
BDRS	Clinician or trained rater	Specific to bipolar depression	Berk *et al.*, 2008	35
		Includes items that are more common in bipolar vs. unipolar depression		
		Very limited use in bipolar clinical trials		
HAM-D	Clinician or trained rater	Most bipolar clinical trials use 17-item version	Silverstone, 2001	15,530
		Developed for MDD		
		International recommended thresholds for bipolar depression trials entry		
		Heavily influenced by physical symptoms		
IDS-C30	Clinician or trained rater	Available in self-rated version as well as clinician version	Calabrese *et al.*, 2010	587
		Administration time of 30 minutes may be longer than the MADRS		
MADRS	Clinician or trained rater	10-items	Tohen *et al.*, 2012	5017
		Developed for MDD		
		Minimal focus on physical symptoms		
		Most popular depression scale in recent bipolar depression clinical trials		
QIDS	Patient-rated	Drawn from the longer IDS	Calabrese *et al.*, 2010	519
		Developed for MDD		
		Can be completed in under 10 minutes		

BDRS: Bipolar Depression Rating Scale; HAM-D: Hamilton Depression Rating Scale; IDS-C30: Inventory of Depressive Symptomatology-30-Item Clinician Version; MADRS: Montgomery Äsberg Depression Rating Scale; MDD: major depressive disorder; QIDS: Quick Inventory of Depressive Symptomatology.

medications have received new U.S. Food and Drug Administration (FDA) indications for acute and maintenance treatment of bipolar depression and mania. The cumulative body of bipolar trials, which include a number of landmark studies, has facilitated consensus on what are critical outcome measurements for efficacy and effectiveness for treatments of people with BD. As noted in Table 9.3,

Table 9.3 Bipolar Remission in Clinical Trials

Remission	Definitions Used in Clinical Trials	Representative Clinical Trial
HAM-D	HAM-D-21 $\leq$ 8	Tohen *et al.*, 2006: olanzapine 48 wks
	HAM-D-17 $\leq$ 5 or $\leq$7	ISBD Task Force: Tohen *et al.*, 2009
MADRS	$\leq$12	Tohen *et al.*, 2003: olanzapine + fluoxetine 8 wks
	$\leq$12	Calabrese *et al.*, 2005: BOLDER I 8 wks
	$\leq$12	Berwaerts *et al.*, 2012: paliperidone ER
	$\leq$12	Suppes *et al.*, 2009: quetiapine 104 wks
	$\leq$12	Young *et al.*, 2010a: quetiapine 8 wks
	$\leq$13 for 26 wks	Keck *et al.*, 2007: aripiprazole 100 wks
	$\leq$12 for 12 wks	Yatham *et al.*, 2013: aripiprazole 52 wks
	$\leq$12 (partial)	Tohen *et al.*, 2012: olanzapine for 6 wks
	$\leq$8 (full)	
	$\leq$5 or $\leq$7	ISBD Task Force: Tohen *et al.*, 2009
YMRS	$\leq$12	Tohen *et al.*, 2006: olanzapine 48 wks
	$\leq$12	Berwaerts *et al.*, 2012: paliperidone ER
	$\leq$12	Suppes *et al.*, 2009: quetiapine 104 wks
	$\leq$10 for 26 wks	Keck *et al.*, 2007: aripiprazole 100 wks
	$\leq$12 for 12 wks	Yatham *et al.*, 2013: aripiprazole 52 wks
	$\leq$12 $\times$ 4 wks	Weisler *et al.*, 2011: quetiapine 104 wks
	$\leq$8	Gopal *et al.*, 2005: risperdal 3 wks
	$\leq$12 or $\leq$7 during and end point	Gopal *et al.*, 2005: risperdal 3 wks
	$\leq$8 or $<$5	ISBD Task Force: Tohen *et al.*, 2009
MRS	$\leq$11	Bowden *et al.*, 2000: divalproex vs. lithium 12 months
	$\leq$12	ISBD Task Force: Tohen *et al.*, 2009
CGI-BD	=1	Post *et al.*, 2006: mood switch 10 wks
	$\leq$2	ISBD Task Force: Tohen *et al.*, 2009
IDS-C30	$<$12	Post *et al.*, 2006: mood switch 10 wks
	$<$12	Frye *et al.*, 2007: modafinil 6 wks

CGI-BD-S: Clinical Global Impression-Bipolar Disorder-Severity of Illness Scale; HAM-D: Hamilton Depression Rating Scale; IDS-C30: Inventory of Depressive Symptomatology-30-Item Clinician Version; ISBD: International Society for Bipolar Disorder; MADRS: Montgomery Äsberg Depression Rating Scale; MRS: Mania Rating Scale; YMRS: Young Mania Rating Scale; wks: weeks.

consensus in standardizing definition of response, remission, relapse, recovery, and recurrence using objective, rating scale-based measurements, have been summarized in the International Society for Bipolar Disorder (ISBD) Task Force report on the nomenclature of course and outcome in BD (Tohen *et al.*, 2009). While a rating scale can of course never capture the full experience that a patient may have in response to a given treatment, it does provide a benchmark to try to evaluate the relative merits of therapies for an individual or groups of individuals.

Bipolar Response using Rating Scales

Response is generally defined as a 50% or more reduction in baseline severity in clinical trials. As qualitative change is partially dependent on an individual's initial severity, the proportion or percent of response may or may not have clinical or personal meaningful significance. Commonly used scales to measure 50% or greater improvement include YMRS, MRS, CGI-BP MADRS, HAM-D, IDS, and BDRS. The ISBD Task Force has proposed to ascribe provisional response when the response criterion is first met, and amend to definite response when the response criterion is still met at the end of 2–4 weeks.

Bipolar Remission using Rating Scales

Remission is defined as the absence or near absence of the signs and symptoms of a treating condition. Unlike response that measures relative change in symptoms from baseline, remission implies absolute resolving of pre-existing symptoms and signs. Patients may have syndromal remission (referring to remission of each of core criterion symptom domains), symptomatic remission (referring to total score threshold as in most clinical trials), sustained remission (referring to remission for predefined period of time), partial remission (referring to having more than minimal symptoms), or full remission (referring to having no more than minimal symptoms). Commonly used scales to evaluate remission include the Patient Health Questionnaire (PHQ-9), QIDS-C16, YMRS, and MRS. Table 9.3 identifies representative clinical trials that use rating scales to identify bipolar remission.

Bipolar Relapse, Recurrence, and Recovery using Rating Scales

Relapse is defined as a return of an episode of index of episode of depression or mania in clinical trials, while recurrence as the appearance of a new episode of depression or mania. Recovery is defined as sustained remission of the last mood episode; however, it does not imply recovery from illness given the chronic, and waxing and waning nature, of BD. Consensus posits that relapse occurs during the continuing phase of treatment after remission while recurrence occurs during the maintenance phase of treatment after recovery (i.e., sustained remission of period of time). As a point of reference, the duration of continuation treatment in unipolar major depressive disorder is widely accepted as 6 months after initial remission, while the maintenance phase begins after sustained remission of 6 months (i.e., recovery) (Furukawa *et al.*, 2008; Moller, Riedel & Seemuller, 2011). However, unlike unipolar major depressive disorder, the natural or expected course of episode of BD is not well defined and may vary depending on the index episode of mania, depression, or mixed status. While there is no clear consensus on what constitutes the duration of the continuation phase of treatment, for operational purposes, the ISBD Task Force has recommended an 8-week duration to define relapse and recurrence (i.e., relapse occurs within 8 weeks of remission, and recurrence occurs after 8 weeks of remission). Table 9.4 illustrates multidimensional bipolar outcomes as measured by rating scales in representative clinical trials.

Table 9.4   Defining Multidimensional Bipolar Outcome using Rating Scales

Scales	Remission	Relapse	Recurrence	Representative Clinical Trial
YMRS HAM-D-21	YMRS ≤ 12 and HAM-D ≤ 8 for 2 consecutive wks during 6–12 wks open-label acute treatment		Symptomatic relapse into any mood episode defined as YMRS score ≥ 15, or HAM-D score ≥ 15, or hospitalization	Tohen *et al.*, 2006 48 wks
MRS DSS GAS SADS-C	MRS ≤ 11 and DSS ≤ 13, and GAS ≥ 60 for 2 consecutive visits during 3 months' acute treatment		MRS ≥ 16 or requiring hospitalization. DSS ≥ 25 requiring antidepressant use or premature discontinuation	Bowden *et al.*, 2000 12 months
GAF QoL based on EuroQol (EQ-5D)	Not having an acute episode during 4–8 wks of run-in phase		New intervention (drug treatment or admission) for an emerging mood episode based on clinical diagnosis	Geddes *et al.*, 2010 24 months
CGI-S HAM-D MRS CGI-I GAS	CGI-S ≤ 3 for 4 wks during 8–16 wks of run-in phase	Relapsed to index mood episode within 90 or 180 days of randomization	The need of intervention for any mood episode	Calabrese *et al.*, 2003 Bowden *et al.*, 2003 76 wks
CDRS-R YMRS CGAS	CDRS-R ≤ 40, and YMRS ≤ 12.5, and CGAS ≥ 51		Premature discontinuation for treatment of emerging symptoms	Findling *et al.*, 2005 76 wks

(Continued...)

Table 9.4 Defining Multidimensional Bipolar Outcome using Rating Scales (Continued)

Scales	Remission	Relapse	Recurrence	Representative Clinical Trial
YMRS MADRS CGI-S	Maintained response during 3 wks open-label oral risperidone and 26 wks open-label long-acting injectable risperidone		YMRS score > 12, MADRS > 12, or CGI-S > 4 at any visit; or episode meeting clinical diagnosis, or new interventions	Quiroz *et al.*, 2010 24 months
YMRS MADRS	YMRS ≤ 12, MADRS ≤ 12 for 4 wks		YMRS score ≥ 20, MADRS ≥ 20 for 2 assessments, or need for intervention for any mood episode	Weisler *et al.*, 2011 104 wks
YMRS MADRS CGI-BP-S	YMRS ≤ 12 and MADRS ≤ 12) for each of last 3 wks during 12 wks of continuation treatment phase		YMRS ≥ 15 and CGI-BP-S ≥ 4 for mania; YMRS < 15, MADRS ≥ 16 and CGI-BP-S ≥ 4 for depression; or need for intervention for any mood episode	Berwaerts *et al.*, 2012 1200 days
YMRS MADRS	YMRS ≤ 12 and MADRS ≤ 12 for four consecutive visits spanning at least 12 wks		YMRS ≥ 20 or MADRS ≥ 20 at two visits; or need for intervention for any mood episode	Suppes *et al.*, 2009 104 wks
YMRS MADRS	YMRS ≤ 10 and MADRS ≤ 13 for 6 wks then 26 wks		Hospitalization or requiring medications for a mood episode	Keck *et al.*, 2007 100 wks
YMRS MADRS	YMRS and MADRS ≤ 12 for 12 consecutive wks		YMRS > 16, MADRS > 16; hospitalization for a mood episode	Yatham *et al.*, 2013 52 wks
YMRS MADRS	YMRS and MADRS ≤ 12 for four visits for total of wks		YMRS ≥ 20, or MADRS ≥ 20 at two consecutive visits, or need for interventions for a mood episode	Vieta *et al.*, 2008 104 wks
CGI-BP-S MADRS YMRS	CGI-BP-S score ≤ 2 for 2 months as sustained remission	Measures include changes in MADRS, YMRS, Beck Scale for Suicide Ideation		Nierenberg *et al.*, 2013 6 months
CGI-I MRS MADRS	CGI-I ≤ 3 for 8 wks, then enter into phase II continuing treatment	MRS ≥ 18, MADRS ≥ 18 x two visits or intervention to a mood episode		Bowden *et al.*, 2010 6 months

Table 9.4 Defining Multidimensional Bipolar Outcome using Rating Scales (Continued)

Scales	Remission	Relapse	Recurrence	Representative Clinical Trial
SUM-D	≤2 syndromal features of mania, hypomania, or depression for ≥ 8 wks (sustained remission)			Nierenberg *et al.*, 2006
SUM-M				Sachs *et al.*, 2007
MADRS				Miklowitz *et al.*, 2007
YMRS				26 wks
MADRS	MADRS ≤ 12 (partial remission), and MADRS ≤ 8 (full remission)		Recovery is defined as MADRS ≤ 12 for ≥ 4 wks of treatment plus completion of the 6-wk acute phase	Tohen *et al.*, 2012 6 wks *Task Force recommendation

CDRS-R: Children's Depression Rating Scale-Revised; CGAS: Children's Global Assessment Scale; CGI-BD-S: Clinical Global Impression-Bipolar Disorder-Severity of Illness; CGI-I: Clinical Global Impression – Global Improvement; CGI-S: Clinical Global Impression-Severity; DSS: Depressive Syndrome Scale; EQ-5D: European Quality of Life Index; GAF: Global Assessment Function; GAS: Global Assessment Scale; HAM-D: Hamilton Rating Scale for Depression; MADRS: Montgomery Åsberg Depression Rating Scale; MRS: Mania Rating Scale; QoL: Quality of life; SADS-C: Schedule of Affective Disorders and Schizophrenia – Change Version; SUM-D: Sum all associated depressive symptom scores; SUM-M: Sum all associated manic symptom scores; wks: weeks; YMRS: Young Mania Rating Scale.

Rating Scales to Assess Other Important Dimensions of Clinical Outcome among Bipolar Patients in Clinical Trials

BD is a complex condition with impairments in multiple domains involving mood symptoms, cognition, behavior, and function. Thus, comprehensive outcome measures of BD in clinical trials should include not only elements of severity of symptoms, duration of response, and remission, but also function. The importance of including a functional measure in clinical trials is highlighted in the McLean-Harvard first-episode mania study (Tohen *et al.*, 2003). In this study, Tohen *et al.* (2003) prospectively followed a cohort of 173 subjects who were hospitalized due to the first episode of mania, and found that by 2 years, despite 98% of the cohort achieving syndromal recovery, only 72% achieved symptomatic recovery, and 43% achieved functional recovery. Though most clinical trials have focused on measuring mood components in primary outcome measures, function assessment has increasingly been included in secondary outcome measures. Commonly used scales include the Global Assessment of Functioning scale (GAF), the 36-item Short-Form Health Survey (SF-36), the World Health Organization Quality of Life (WHO-QoL), the Quality of Life Enjoyment and Satisfaction Questionnaire (Q-LES-Q), and the European Quality of Life Index (EQ-5D). All these are nondisease-specific instruments and predominantly were designed for monitoring health levels in whole communities (Endicott *et al.*, 1993; EuroQol Group, 1990; McHorney, Ware & Raczek, 1993; Trompenaars *et al.*, 2005). These scales were mostly used as continuing variables for mean change

(Bowden *et al.*, 2000; Calabrese *et al.*, 2003, 2005; Geddes *et al.*, 2010; Namjoshi *et al.*, 2002; Nierenberg *et al.*, 2006, 2013). In one study, the authors suggest that a cutoff score of 50 or greater for standardized physical component and 49 or greater for the SF-36 standardized mental component of the SF-36 and 0.88 or greater for the EQ-5D index approximates a CGI-BP definition of remission (i.e., CGI-BP $\leq$ 2 as 1 being normal/not at all being ill and 2 being borderline mentally ill) (Subero *et al.*, 2013).

Since most currently available scales were not specifically developed to assess areas of functional impairment in BD, the Functioning Assessment Short-Test (FAST) was developed and validated to assess six specific domains of psychosocial function in patients with BD: autonomy, occupational and cognitive functioning, financial issues, interpersonal relationships, and leisure time. The scale requires approximately 5 minutes to complete, and it can be used to measure the change in the course of interventions. The FAST has 24 items with overall score ranges from 0 to 72, with higher scores indicating greater disability. The authors suggest a cutoff value of less than 11 as indicating functional remission (Rosa *et al.*, 2007). FAST was used in a randomized controlled trial testing effectiveness of collaborative care program in comparison to care as usual. The study assessed 12 months of psychosocial functioning (measured by FAST), symptoms, and quality of life in patients with BD (van der Voort *et al.*, 2011).

RATING SCALES IN BIPOLAR POPULATIONS ACROSS THE LIFESPAN
Older Individuals with Bipolar Disorder

Epidemiologic studies suggest that BD spectrum illness affects approximately 0.5–1.0% of adults above the age of 60 (Kessing & Nilsson, 2003; Kessler *et al.*, 2005; Unutzer *et al.*, 1998). While BD becomes less common with age (it is approximately one-third as common as it is in younger populations), bipolar illness is present in 6% of geriatric psychiatry outpatient visits and 8–10% of geriatric inpatient admissions (Depp & Jeste, 2004). Given increasing lifespan and changes in global demographics, it is anticipated that the absolute numbers of older people with BD will also increase. There is remarkably little information available regarding standardized ratings of either manic or depressive symptoms in geriatric BD (Sajatovic *et al.*, 2011b; Young, Peasley-Miklus & Shulberg, 2007; Young *et al.*, 2010b). As with mixed-age patients with BD, the YMRS is the most common mania severity measure in recently published reports on geriatric bipolar clinical trials (Sajatovic, Calabrese & Mullen, 2008a; Sajatovic *et al.*, 2008b; 2011a; Young *et al.*, 2010a). For depressive symptoms, potential limitations of the HAM-D in geriatric populations include its heavy reliance on somatic symptoms that could be potentially misleading in elderly subpopulations with medical comorbidity (Berk *et al.*, 2004; Linden *et al.*, 1995). Older people with BD have multiple medical comorbidities, in particular type II diabetes, respiratory and cardiovascular conditions, and other endocrine abnormalities. A mean of three or four medical conditions appears to be the norm (Lala & Sajatovic, 2012). However, in spite of its shortcomings in medically complex older people, the HAM-D is still widely used in geriatric bipolar clinical trials. Reports focused on late-life BD have used either the HAM-D (Gildengers *et al.*, 2005; Sajatovic *et al.*, 2008b) or the MADRS (Montgomery & Äsberg, 1979) to assess depressive symptoms (Sajatovic *et al.*, 2008a; 2011a). One clinical trial in geriatric bipolar patients (mean age 68.9 years, standard deviation 7.1) found that bipolar depression symptoms severity measures using the MADRS and HAM-D were highly correlated (Sajatovic *et al.*, 2011b).

Within the older population, manic psychopathology can present in people with neurodegenerative conditions/dementia, as well as in cognitively intact individuals. Instruments designed to document various behavioral abnormalities in patients with dementia may include manic signs and symptoms; examples are the Dementia Signs and Symptoms Scale (Loreck, Bylsma & Folstein, 1994) and the Neuropsychiatric Inventory (NPI) (Cummings *et al.*, 1994).

Important considerations in late-life BD that may be a focus in clinical trials involving older people with BD is the presence of medical burden and cognitive impairments that may occur even in geriatric patients who do not have a clinical diagnosis of dementia. Geriatric bipolar clinical trials (Sajatovic *et al.*, 2011a; Young *et al.*, 2010b) have assessed overall medical comorbidity with the Cumulative Illness Rating Scale – Geriatric Version (CIRS-G) (Miller *et al.*, 1992) and cognitive status with the Mini-Mental State Examination (MMSE) (Folstein, Folstein & McHugh, 1975). These brief standardized assessments might be supplemented with more specific medical assessments such as cardiovascular risk or finer-grained neuropsychological evaluation depending on the population focus.

Children with Bipolar Disorder

Pediatric BD resembles BD as seen in adults. BD in children may start at very young ages and can be associated with such negative outcomes as school under-performance or failure, family distress, and a wide range of psychosocial problems (Carter *et al.*, 2003; Geller *et al.*, 2008; Leverich *et al.*, 2007; Lin *et al.*, 2006; Perlis *et al.*, 2004). The symptom presentation of BD in children is characterized by extreme mood lability, mixed states, extensive comorbidity, and rapid cycling, which distinguish the pediatric bipolarity from its adult counterpart (Pavuluri, Birmaher & Naylor, 2005). Fortunately, the evidence base derived from clinical trials in pediatric BD is growing (Washburn, West & Heil, 2011), although the majority of clinical trials in bipolar children are mania studies.

The Parent – General Behavior Inventory (P-GBI) (Youngstrom *et al.*, 2001, 2005, 2008) is an adaptation of a well-validated instrument for screening for mood disorder in adults. The P-GBI contains 73 Likert-type items rated on a 0–3 continuum (0 = 'Never or Hardly Ever' and 3 = 'Very often or Almost Constantly'), with higher scores indicating greater illness severity

(Youngstrom *et al.*, 2001). Youngstrom and colleagues have developed a 10-item version of the P-GBI (Youngstrom *et al.*, 2008) intended as a screening tool for pediatric mania.

As with mixed-age populations, clinical treatment studies in pediatric bipolar mania frequently use the YMRS to assess change over time in manic symptoms (Findling *et al.*, 2009; Mankoski *et al.*, 2011; Pavuluri *et al.*, 2010). The YMRS has been validated in pediatric bipolar patients (Youngstrom *et al.*, 2002). Reflecting the need for a parental involvement and input to assess treatment effects in children with mania, the Child Mania Rating Scale (CMRS-P) is a 21-item parent mania rating scale (Henry *et al.*, 2008; Pavuluri *et al.*, 2006). Items are drawn from the DSM-IV criteria for a manic episode and are age-specific. Items on the CMRS-P are considered to be a problem only they are causing impairment, deviate from norms for the child's age, and have been causing a problem in the last month. Items are scored on a 4-point continuum (0 = never/rare, 1 = sometimes, 2 = often, and 3 = very often). The scale takes approximately 10–15 minutes to complete. Compared to clinician-administered instruments, the CMRS-P has an internal consistency reliability of 0.96 and shows sensitivity and specificity for differentiating pediatric mania from other disorders and no disorder (Pavuluri *et al.*, 2006). A score of 20 differentiates children with BD from healthy controls and from children with attention deficit hyperactive disorder (ADHD) and has been suggested as a pediatric mania remission cutoff. There is also a brief, 10-item version of the CMRS-P (Brief CMRS-P). A validation study on the Brief CMRS-P found that using a score of 10 as a cutoff point had high sensitivity and specificity for differentiating pediatric bipolar mania from ADHD (Henry *et al.*, 2008).

FUTURE DIRECTIONS IN APPLICATIONS OF RATING SCALES IN BIPOLAR CLINICAL TRIALS

Given the increased globalization of clinical research studies, the use of standardized scales will help to facilitate comparison of treatments and outcomes. In addition, rating scales used in clinical trials can be expected to adapt to emerging agendas. For example, a newly developed DSM-5 has "softened" the diagnosis of mixed bipolar states, and there is now a course specifier for mixed BD (American Psychiatric Association, 2013), which may become a greater focus in bipolar clinical trials. Particularly relevant to mixed states, use of a rating scale that assesses bipolar manic, depressive, and mixed symptoms simultaneously and in one scale is especially attractive. The Bipolar Inventory of Signs and Symptoms (BISS) scale developed by Bowden and colleagues (Bowden *et al.*, 2007; Gonzalez *et al.*, 2008; Singh *et al.*, 2013; Thompson *et al.*, 2010) is a semistructured rating scale developed to assess a broad spectrum of reported and observed behaviors seen in individuals with BD. There are 44 items scored on a 0–4 continuum (0 = not at all, 4 = severe) with descriptive anchors for each score. The BISS yields a total score, depression and mania scores, as well as item scores. Reliability and validity is good

(Bowden *et al.*, 2007; Gonzalez *et al.*, 2008). The BISS is able to differentiate depressed, mixed, and manic/hypomanic states from recovered status as well as being able to identify primary bipolar clinical states (Singh *et al.*, 2013). A small set of symptom items on the BISS (mainly manic and anxiety components) have the potential to identify individuals with bipolar mixed states (Singh *et al.*, 2013). The BISS supports the clinical assumption that overall bipolar symptom severity may be greater in bipolar mixed episodes compared with purely depressed or manic states (Singh *et al.*, 2013).

Other directions for the future include a growing focus on patient-centered outcomes that includes input and perceived value by people with BD. Self-rated scales are likely to become increasingly an important primary or secondary outcome. Additionally, there is ongoing need to make clinical trials cost and time efficient. Approaches that minimize steps and efforts such as online rating scale item entry and immediate centralized data collection are likely to become increasingly common in the future. Finally, novel analytic methods that merge data from multiple randomized controlled trials (Leucht *et al.*, 2012) will extend our ability to interpret clinical trial findings, but these types of analyses appear most robust when there is relative homogeneity across trials, such as use of the same rating scales to assess outcomes and tight consensus on definitions of treatment response as well as criteria for relapse and recovery. Thus, there will be an increasing need to standardize outcome measurement approaches on an international level.

REFERENCES

Adler, M., Liberg, B., Andersson, S., et al. (2008). Development and validation of the affective self-rating scale for manic, depressive, and mixed affective states. *Nordic Journal of Psychiatry, 62*(2), 130–135.

Ahearn, E. P., & Carroll, B. J. (1996). Short-term variability of mood ratings in unipolar and bipolar depressed patients. *Journal of Affective Disorders, 36*(3–4), 107–115.

Altman, E. G., Hedeker, D., Peterson, J. L., & Davis, J. M. (1997). The altman self-rating mania scale. *Biological Psychiatry, 42*(10), 948–955.

Altman, E. G., Hedeker, D. R., Janicak, P. G., et al. (1994). The Clinician-Administered Rating Scale for Mania (CARS-M): Development, reliability, and validity. *Biological Psychiatry, 36*(2), 124–134.

American Psychiatric Association. (2000). *Diagnostic and statistical manual of mental disorders: DSM-IV-TR*. American Psychiatric Publishing, Inc.

American Psychiatric Association. (2013). *Diagnostic and statistical manual of mental disorders: DSM-5*. American Psychiatric Publishing, Inc.

Äsberg, M., Montgomery, S. A., Perris, C., et al. (1978). A comprehensive psychopathological rating scale. *Acta Psychiatrica Scandinavica Supplementum, 271*, 5–27.

Bagby, R. M., Ryder, A. G., Schuller, D. R., et al. (2004). The Hamilton depression rating scale: Has the gold standard become a lead weight? *American Journal of Psychiatry, 161*(12), 2163–2177.

Bauer, M. S., Vojta, C., Kinosian, B., et al. (2000). The Internal state scale: Replication of its discriminating abilities in a multisite, public sector sample. *Bipolar Disorders, 2*(4), 340–346.

Bech, P. (2002). The Bech-Rafaelsen mania scale in clinical trials of therapies for bipolar disorder: A 20-year review of its use as an outcome measure. *CNS Drugs, 16*(1), 47–63.

Bech, P., Bolwig, T. G., Kramp, P., et al. (1979). The bech-rafaelsen mania scale and the Hamilton depression scale. *Acta Psychiatrica Scandinavica*, *59*(4), 420–430.

Beck, A. T., & Steer, R. A. (1993). *Manual for the beck depression inventory*. San Antonio: Psychological Corporation.

Beck, A. T., Steer, R. A., & Garbing, M. G. (1988). Psychometric properties of the Beck Depression Inventory: Twenty-five years of evaluation. *Clinical Psychology Review*, *8*, 77–100.

Beigel, A., Murphy, D. L., & Bunney, W. E. (1971). The manic-state rating scale: Scale construction, reliability, and validity. *Archives of General Psychiatry*, *25*, 256–262.

Benazzi, F., Berk, M., Frye, M. A., et al. (2009). Olanzapine/fluoxetine combination for the treatment of mixed depression in bipolar I disorder: A post hoc analysis. *Journal of Clinical Psychiatry*, *70*(10), 1424–1431.

Berk, M., Copolov, D. L., Dean, O., et al. (2008). N-acetyl cysteine for depressive symptoms in bipolar disorder – a double-blind randomized placebo-controlled trial. *Biological Psychiatry*, *64*(6), 468–475.

Berk, M., Malhi, G. S., Cahill, C., et al. (2007). The Bipolar Depression Rating Scale (BDRS): Its development, validation and utility. *Bipolar Disorders*, *9*(6), 571–579.

Berk, M., Malhi, G. S., Mitchell, P. B., et al. (2004). Scale matters: The need for a Bipolar Depression Rating Scale (BDRS). *Acta Psychiatrica Scandinavica Supplementum*, *422*, 39–45.

Berwaerts, J., Melkote, R., Nuamah, I., et al. (2012). A randomized, placebo- and active-controlled study of paliperidone extended-release as maintenance treatment in patients with bipolar I disorder after an acute manic or mixed episode. *Journal of Affective Disorders*, *138*(3), 247–258.

Blackburn, I. M., Loudon, J. B., & Ashworth, C. M. (1977). A new scale for measuring mania. *Psychological Medicine*, *7*(3), 453–458.

Bowden, C. L., Brugger, A. M., Swann, A. C., et al. (1994). Efficacy of divalproex vs lithium and placebo in the treatment of mania. The Depakote Mania Study Group. *JAMA*, *271*(12), 918–924.

Bowden, C. L., Calabrese, J. R., McElroy, S. L., et al. (2000). A randomized, placebo-controlled 12-month trial of divalproex and lithium in treatment of outpatients with bipolar I disorder. Divalproex Maintenance Study Group. *Archives of General Psychiatry*, *57*(5), 481–489.

Bowden, C. L., Calabrese, J. R., Sachs, G., et al. (2003). A placebo-controlled 18-month trial of lamotrigine and lithium maintenance treatment in recently manic or hypomanic patients with bipolar I disorder. *Archives of General Psychiatry*, *60*(4), 392–400.

Bowden, C. L., Singh, V., Thompson, P., et al. (2007). Development of the bipolar inventory of symptoms scale. *Acta Psychiatrica Scandinavica*, *116*(3), 189–194.

Bowden, C. L., Vieta, E., Ice, K. S., et al. (2010). Ziprasidone plus a mood stabilizer in subjects with bipolar I disorder: A 6-month, randomized, placebo-controlled, double-blind trial. *Journal of Clinical Psychiatry*, *71*(2), 130–137.

Cahill, C. M., Malhi, G. S., Berk, M., et al. (2005). Exploration of symptomatic differences between bipolar and unipolar depression. *Australian and New Zealand Journal of Psychiatry*, *39*(2), 48.

Calabrese, J. R., Bowden, C. L., Sachs, G., et al. (2003). A placebo-controlled 18-month trial of lamotrigine and lithium maintenance treatment in recently depressed patients with bipolar I disorder. *Journal of Clinical Psychiatry*, *64*(9), 1013–1024.

Calabrese, J. R., Bowden, C. L., Sachs, G. S., et al. (1999). A double-blind placebo-controlled study of lamotrigine monotherapy in outpatients with bipolar I depression. Lamictal 602 Study Group. *Journal of Clinical Psychiatry*, *60*(2), 79–88.

Calabrese, J. R., Huffman, R. F., White, R. L., et al. (2008). Lamotrigine in the acute treatment of bipolar depression: Results of five double-blind, placebo-controlled clinical trials. *Bipolar Disorders*, *10*(2), 323–333.

Calabrese, J. R., Keck, P. E., Jr., Macfadden, W., et al. (2005). A randomized, double-blind, placebo-controlled trial of quetiapine in the treatment of bipolar I or II depression. *American Journal of Psychiatry*, *162*(7), 1351–1360.

Calabrese, J. R., Ketter, T. A., Youakim, J. M., et al. (2010). Adjunctive armodafinil for major depressive episodes associated with bipolar I disorder: A randomized, multicenter, double-blind, placebo-controlled, proof-of-concept study. *Journal of Clinical Psychiatry*, *71*(10), 1363–1370.

Carter, T. D., Mundo, E., Parikh, S. V., et al. (2003). Early age at onset as a risk factor for poor outcome of bipolar disorder. *Journal of Psychiatric Research*, *37*(4), 297–303.

Craddock, N., Jones, I., Kirov, G., et al. (2004). The Bipolar Affective Disorder Dimension Scale (BADDS) – a dimensional scale for rating lifetime psychopathology in bipolar spectrum disorders. *BMC Psychiatry*, *4*, 19.

Cummings, J. L., Mega, M., Gray, K., et al. (1994). The Neuropsychiatric Inventory: Comprehensive assessment of psychopathology in dementia. *Neurology*, *44*(12), 2308–2314.

Depp, C. A., & Jeste, D. V. (2004). Bipolar disorder in older adults: A critical review. *Bipolar Disorders*, *6*(5), 343–367.

Depue, R. A., Krauss, S., Spoont, M. R., et al. (1989). General behavior inventory identification of unipolar and bipolar affective conditions in a nonclinical university population. *Journal of Abnormal Psychology*, *98*(2), 117–126.

Dorz, S., Borgherini, G., Conforti, D., et al. (2003). Depression in inpatients: Bipolar vs unipolar. *Psychological Reports*, *92*(3 Pt 1), 1031–1039.

Endicott, J., Nee, J., Harrison, W., et al. (1993). Quality of life enjoyment and satisfaction questionnaire: A new measure. *Psychopharmacology Bulletin*, *29*(2), 321–326.

Endicott, J., & Spitzer, R. L. (1978). A diagnostic interview: The schedule for affective disorders and schizophrenia. *Archives of General Psychiatry*, *35*(7), 837–844.

EuroQol Group (1990). EuroQol – a new facility for the measurement of health-related quality of life. *Health Policy (Amsterdam, Netherlands)*, *16*(3), 199–208.

Findling, R. L., McNamara, N. K., Youngstrom, E. A., et al. (2005). Double-blind 18-month trial of lithium versus divalproex maintenance treatment in pediatric bipolar disorder. *Journal of the American Academy of Child and Adolescent Psychiatry*, *44*(5), 409–417.

Findling, R. L., Nyilas, M., Forbes, R. A., et al. (2009). Acute treatment of pediatric bipolar I disorder, manic or mixed episode, with aripiprazole: A randomized, double-blind, placebo-controlled study. *Journal of Clinical Psychiatry*, *70*(10), 1441–1451.

Folstein, M. F., Folstein, S. E., & McHugh, P. R. (1975). "Mini-Mental State". A practical method for grading the cognitive state of patients for the clinician. *Journal of Psychiatric Research*, *12*(3), 189–198.

Fountoulakis, K. N., Kasper, S., Andreassen, O., et al. (2012). Efficacy of pharmacotherapy in bipolar disorder: A report by the WPA section on pharmacopsychiatry. *European Archives of Psychiatry and Clinical Neuroscience*, *262*(Suppl. 1), 1–48.

Freeman, T. W., Clothier, J. L., Pazzaglia, P., et al. (1992). A double-blind comparison of valproate and lithium in the treatment of acute mania. *American Journal of Psychiatry*, *149*(1), 108–111.

Frye, M. A., Grunze, H., Suppes, T., et al. (2007). A placebo-controlled evaluation of adjunctive modafinil in the treatment of bipolar depression. *American Journal of Psychiatry*, *164*(8), 1242–1249.

Furukawa, T. A., Fujita, A., Harai, H., et al. (2008). Definitions of recovery and outcomes of major depression: Results from a 10-year follow-up. *Acta Psychiatrica Scandinavica*, *117*(1), 35–40.

Galvao, F., Sportiche, S., Lambert, J., et al. (2013). Clinical differences between unipolar and bipolar depression: Interest of BDRS (Bipolar Depression Rating Scale). *Comprehensive Psychiatry*, *54*(6), 605–610.

Garza-Trevino, E. S., Overall, J. E., & Hollister, L. E. (1992). Verapamil versus lithium in acute mania. *American Journal of Psychiatry*, *149*(1), 121–122.

Geddes, J. R., Goodwin, G. M., Rendell, J., et al. (2010). Lithium plus valproate combination therapy versus monotherapy for relapse prevention in bipolar I disorder (BALANCE): A randomised open-label trial. *Lancet*, *375*(9712), 385–395.

Geller, B., Tillman, R., Bolhofner, K., et al. (2008). Child bipolar I disorder: Prospective continuity with adult bipolar I disorder; characteristics of second and third episodes; predictors of 8-year outcome. *Archives of General Psychiatry*, *65*(10), 1125–1133.

Ghaemi, S. N., Miller, C. J., Berv, D. A., et al. (2005). Sensitivity and specificity of a new bipolar spectrum diagnostic scale. *Journal of Affective Disorders*, *84*(2–3), 273–277.

Gildengers, A. G., Mulsant, B. H., Begley, A. E., et al. (2005). A pilot study of standardized treatment in geriatric bipolar disorder. *American Journal of Geriatric Psychiatry*, *13*(4), 319–323.

Gonzalez, J. M., Bowden, C. L., Katz, M. M., et al. (2008). Development of the bipolar inventory of symptoms scale: Concurrent validity, discriminant validity and retest reliability. *International Journal of Methods in Psychiatric Research*, *17*(4), 198–209.

Goodwin, G. M., Anderson, I., Arango, C., et al. (2008). ECNP consensus meeting. Bipolar depression. Nice, March 2007. *European Neuropsychopharmacology*, *18*(7), 535–549.

Gopal, S., Steffens, D. C., Kramer, M. L., et al. (2005). Symptomatic remission in patients with bipolar mania: Results from a double-blind, placebo-controlled trial of risperidone monotherapy. *Journal of Clinical Psychiatry*, *66*(8), 1016–1020.

Grunze, H., Erfurth, A., Marcuse, A., et al. (1999). Tiagabine appears not to be efficacious in the treatment of acute mania. *Journal of Clinical Psychiatry*, *60*(11), 759–762.

Guy, W. (1976). *ECDEU assessment manual for psychopharmacology. publication no. (ADM)*. Rockville, MD: U.S. Department of Health, Education, and Welfare (DHEW).

Hamilton, M. (1960). A rating scale for depression. *Journal of Neurology, Neurosurgery, and Psychiatry*, *23*, 56–62.

Hamilton, M. (1967). Development of a rating scale for primary depressive illness. *British Journal of Social and Clinical Psychology*, *6*(4), 278–296.

Hamilton, M. (1976). Hamilton psychiatric rating scale for depression. In W. Guy (Ed.), *ECDEU Assessment manual for psychopharmacology* (pp. 179–192). Washington, DC: US Department of Health, Education, and Welfare.

Hayes, M. H. S., & Patterson, D. G. (1921). Experimental development of the graphic rating method. *Psychological Bulletin*, *18*, 98–99.

Henry, D. B., Pavuluri, M. N., Youngstrom, E., et al. (2008). Accuracy of brief and full forms of the Child Mania Rating Scale. *Journal of Clinical Psychology*, *64*(4), 368–381.

Hirschfeld, R. M. (2002). The Mood Disorder Questionnaire: A simple, patient-rated screening instrument for bipolar disorder. *Primary Care Companion to the Journal of Clinical Psychiatry*, *4*(1), 9–11.

Hirschfeld, R. M., Allen, M. H., McEvoy, J. P., et al. (1999). Safety and tolerability of oral loading divalproex sodium in acutely manic bipolar patients. *Journal of Clinical Psychiatry*, *60*(12), 815–818.

International Review of Psychosis and Bipolar Disorders (IRBD). *Scales and assessment*. (2012). <http://www.irbd.org/scales.php/> Accessed 30.07.14.

Janicak, P. G., Keck, P. E., Jr., et al., Davis, J. M., et al. (2001). A double-blind, randomized, prospective evaluation of the efficacy and safety of risperidone versus haloperidol in the treatment of schizoaffective disorder. *Journal of Clinical Psychopharmacology*, *21*(4), 360–368.

Judd, L. L., Akiskal, H. S., Schettler, P. J., et al. (2002). The long-term natural history of the weekly symptomatic status of bipolar I disorder. *Archives of General Psychiatry*, *59*(6), 530–537.

Judd, L. L., Akiskal, H. S., Schettler, P. J., et al. (2005). Psychosocial disability in the course of bipolar I and II disorders: A prospective, comparative, longitudinal study. *Archives of General Psychiatry*, *62*(12), 1322–1330.

Kalai, A., Wiliams, J. B., Koback, K. A., et al. (2002). The new GRID HAM-D: Pilot testing and international field trials. *International Journal of Neuropsychopharmacology*, *5*, S147–S148.

Katz, M. M., & Itil, T. M. (1974). Video methodology for research in psychopathology and psychopharmacology: Rationale and application. *Archives of General Psychiatry*, *31*(2), 204–210.

Keck, P. E., Jr., Calabrese, J. R., McIntyre, R. S., et al. (2007). Aripiprazole monotherapy for maintenance therapy in bipolar I disorder: A 100-week, double-blind study versus placebo. *Journal of Clinical Psychiatry, 68*(10), 1480–1491.

Kessing, L. V., & Nilsson, F. M. (2003). Increased risk of developing dementia in patients with major affective disorders compared to patients with other medical illnesses. *Journal of Affective Disorders, 73*(3), 261–269.

Kessler, R. C., Berglund, P., Demler, O., et al. (2005). Lifetime prevalence and age-of-onset distributions of DSM-IV disorders in the National Comorbidity Survey Replication. *Archives of General Psychiatry, 62*(6), 593–602.

Lala, S. V., & Sajatovic, M. (2012). Medical and psychiatric comorbidities among elderly individuals with bipolar disorder: A literature review. *Journal of Geriatric Psychiatry and Neurology, 25*(1), 20–25.

Lerer, B., Moore, N., Meyendorff, E., et al. (1987). Carbamazepine versus lithium in mania: A double-blind study. *Journal of Clinical Psychiatry, 48*(3), 89–93.

Leucht, S., Tardy, M., Komossa, K., et al. (2012). Antipsychotic drugs versus placebo for relapse prevention in schizophrenia: A systematic review and meta-analysis. *Lancet, 379*(9831), 2063–2071.

Leverich, G. S., Post, R. M., Keck, P. E., Jr., et al. (2007). The poor prognosis of childhood-onset bipolar disorder. *Journal of Pediatrics, 150*(5), 485–490.

Lin, P. I., McInnis, M. G., Potash, J. B., et al. (2006). Clinical correlates and familial aggregation of age at onset in bipolar disorder. *American Journal of Psychiatry, 163*(2), 240–246.

Linden, M., Borchelt, M., Barnow, S., et al. (1995). The impact of somatic morbidity on the Hamilton Depression Rating Scale in the very old. *Acta Psychiatrica Scandinavica, 92*(2), 150–154.

Loreck, D. J., Bylsma, F. W., & Folstein, M. F. (1994). A new scale for comprehensive assessment of psychopathology in Alzheimer's disease. *American Journal of Geriatric Psychiatry, 2*(1), 60–74.

Loudon, J. B., Blackburn, I. M., & Ashworth, C. M. (1977). A study of the symptomatology and course of manic illness using a new scale. *Psychological Medicine, 7*(4), 723–729.

Mankoski, R., Zhao, J., Carson, W. H., et al. (2011). Young Mania Rating Scale line item analysis in pediatric subjects with bipolar I disorder treated with aripiprazole in a short-term, double-blind, randomized study. *Journal of Child and Adolescent Psychopharmacology, 21*(4), 359–364.

McHorney, C. A., Ware, J. E., Jr., & Raczek, A. E. (1993). The MOS 36-Item Short-Form Health Survey (SF-36: II. Psychometric and clinical tests of validity in measuring physical and mental health constructs. *Medical Care, 31*(3), 247–263.

Merikangas, K. R., Akiskal, H. S., Angst, J., et al. (2007). Lifetime and 12-month prevalence of bipolar spectrum disorder in the National Comorbidity Survey Replication. *Archives of General Psychiatry, 64*(5), 543–552.

Miklowitz, D. J., Otto, M. W., Frank, E., et al. (2007). Psychosocial treatments for bipolar depression: A 1-year randomized trial from the systematic treatment enhancement program. *Archives of General Psychiatry, 64*(4), 419–426.

Miller, M. D., Paradis, C. F., Houck, P. R., et al. (1992). Rating chronic medical illness burden in geropsychiatric practice and research: Application of the Cumulative Illness Rating Scale. *Psychiatry Research, 41*(3), 237–248.

Moller, H. J., Riedel, M., & Seemuller, F. (2011). Relapse or recurrence in depression: Why has the cutoff been set at 6 months? *Medicographia, 33*, 125–131.

Montgomery, S., & Asberg, M. (1979). A new depression scale designed to be sensitive to change. *British Journal of Psychiatry, 134*, 382–389.

Montgomery, S., Asberg, M., Jornestedt, L., et al. (1978). Reliability of the CPRS between the disciplines of psychiatry, general practice, nursing and psychology in depressed patients. *Acta Psychiatrica Scandinavica Supplementum, 271*, 29–32.

Murphy, D. L., Beigel, A., Weingartner, H., et al. (1974). The quantitation of manic behavior. *Modern Problems of Pharmacopsychiatry, 7*, 203–220.

Murphy, D. L., Pickar, D., Alterman, I. S., et al. (1982). Methods for the quantitative assessment of depressive and manic behavior. In E. J. Burdock, A. Sudilovsky, &

S. Gershon (Eds.), *The behavior of psychiatric patients* (pp. 355–392). New York: Marcel Dekker.

Namjoshi, M. A., Rajamannar, G., Jacobs, T., et al. (2002). Economic, clinical, and quality-of-life outcomes associated with olanzapine treatment in mania. Results from a randomized controlled trial. *Journal of Affective Disorders, 69*(1–3), 109–118.

Nierenberg, A. A., Friedman, E. S., Bowden, C. L., et al. (2013). Lithium Treatment Moderate-Dose Use Study (LiTMUS) for bipolar disorder: A randomized comparative effectiveness trial of optimized personalized treatment with and without lithium. *The American Journal of Psychiatry, 170*(1), 102–110.

Nierenberg, A. A., Ostacher, M. J., Calabrese, J. R., et al. (2006). Treatment-resistant bipolar depression: A STEP-BD equipoise randomized effectiveness trial of antidepressant augmentation with lamotrigine, inositol, or risperidone. *American Journal of Psychiatry, 163*(2), 210–216.

Overall, J. E., & Gorham, D. R. (1962). The brief psychiatric rating scale. *Psychological Reports, 10*(3), 799–812.

Pavuluri, M. N., Birmaher, B., & Naylor, M. W. (2005). Pediatric bipolar disorder: A review of the past 10 years. *Journal of the American Academy of Child and Adolescent Psychiatry, 44*(9), 846–871.

Pavuluri, M. N., Henry, D. B., Devineni, B., et al. (2006). Child Mania Rating Scale: Development, reliability, and validity. *Journal of the American Academy of Child and Adolescent Psychiatry, 45*(5), 550–560.

Pavuluri, M. N., Henry, D. B., Findling, R. L., et al. (2010). Double-blind randomized trial of risperidone versus divalproex in pediatric bipolar disorder. *Bipolar Disorders, 12*(6), 593–605.

Perlis, R. H., Miyahara, S., Marangell, L. B., et al. (2004). Long-term implications of early onset in bipolar disorder: Data from the first 1000 participants in the Systematic Treatment Enhancement Program for Bipolar Disorder (STEP-BD). *Biological Psychiatry, 55*(9), 875–881.

Petterson, U., Fyro, B., & Sedvall, G. (1973). A new scale for the longitudinal rating of manic states. *Acta Psychiatrica Scandinavica, 49*(3), 248–256.

Picardi, A. (2009). Rating scales in bipolar disorder. *Current Opinion in Psychiatry, 22*(1), 42–49.

Plutchik, R., Platman, S. R., Tilles, R., et al. (1970). Construction and evaluation of a test for measuring mania and depression. *Journal of Clinical Psychology, 26*(4), 499–503.

Post, R. M., Altshuler, L. L., Leverich, G. S., et al. (2006). Mood switch in bipolar depression: Comparison of adjunctive venlafaxine, bupropion and sertraline. *British Journal of Psychiatry, 189*, 124–131.

Quiroz, J. A., Yatham, L. N., Palumbo, J. M., et al. (2010). Risperidone long-acting injectable monotherapy in the maintenance treatment of bipolar I disorder. *Biological Psychiatry, 68*(2), 156–162.

Robinson, L. J., & Ferrier, I. N. (2006). Evolution of cognitive impairment in bipolar disorder: A systematic review of cross-sectional evidence. *Bipolar Disorders, 8*(2), 103–116.

Rosa, A. R., Sanchez-Moreno, J., Martinez-Aran, A., et al. (2007). Validity and reliability of the Functioning Assessment Short Rest (FAST) in bipolar disorder. *Clinical Practice and Epidemiology in Mental Health, 3*, 5.

Rush, A. J., Gullion, C. M., Basco, M. R., et al. (1996). The Inventory of Depressive Symptomatology (IDS): Psychometric properties. *Psychological Medicine, 26*(3), 477–486.

Rush, A. J., Trivedi, M. H., Ibrahim, H. M., et al. (2003). The 16-item Quick Inventory of Depressive Symptomatology (QIDS), Clinician Rating (QIDS-C), and Self-Report (QIDS-SR): A psychometric evaluation in patients with chronic major depression. *Biological Psychiatry, 54*(5), 573–583.

Sachs, G. S., Nierenberg, A. A., Calabrese, J. R., et al. (2007). Effectiveness of adjunctive antidepressant treatment for bipolar depression. *New England Journal of Medicine, 356*(17), 1711–1722.

Sajatovic, M., Calabrese, J. R., & Mullen, J. (2008a). Quetiapine for the treatment of bipolar mania in older adults. *Bipolar Disorders, 10*(6), 662–671.

Sajatovic, M., Coconcea, N., Ignacio, R. V., et al. (2008b). Aripiprazole therapy in 20 older adults with bipolar disorder: A 12-week, open-label trial. *Journal of Clinical Psychiatry*, *69*(1), 41–46.

Sajatovic, M., Gildengers, A., Al Jurdi, R. K., et al. (2011a). Multisite, open-label, prospective trial of lamotrigine for geriatric bipolar depression: A preliminary report. *Bipolar Disorders*, *13*(3), 294–302.

Sajatovic, M., Al Jurdi, R. A., Gildengers, A., et al. (2011b). Depression symptom ratings in geriatric patients with bipolar mania. *International Journal of Geriatric Psychiatry*, *26*(11), 1201–1208.

Sajatovic, M., & Ramirez, L. (2013). *Rating scales in mental health* (3rd ed.). Baltimore, MD: Johns Hopkins Press.

Saricicek, A., Maloney, K., Muralidharan, A., et al. (2011). Levetiracetam in the management of bipolar depression: A randomized, double-blind, placebo-controlled trial. *Journal of Clinical Psychiatry*, *72*(6), 744–750.

Secunda, S. K., Katz, M. M., Swann, A., et al. (1985). Mania. Diagnosis, state measurement and prediction of treatment response. *Journal of Affective Disorders*, *8*(2), 113–121.

Shafti, S. S. (2010). Olanzapine vs. lithium in management of acute mania. *Journal of Affective Disorders*, *122*(3), 273–276.

Shopsin, B., Gershon, S., Thompson, H., et al. (1975). Psychoactive drugs in mania. A controlled comparison of lithium carbonate, chlorpromazine, and haloperidol. *Archives of General Psychiatry*, *32*(1), 34–42.

Shugar, G., Schertzer, S., Toner, B. B., et al. (1992). Development, use, and factor analysis of a self-report inventory for mania. *Comprehensive Psychiatry*, *33*(5), 325–331.

Silverstone, T. (2001). Moclobemide vs. imipramine in bipolar depression: A multicentre double-blind clinical trial. *Acta Psychiatrica Scandinavica*, *104*(2), 104–109.

Singh, V., Bowden, C. L., Gonzalez, J. M., et al. (2013). Discriminating primary clinical states in bipolar disorder with a comprehensive symptom scale. *Acta Psychiatrica Scandinavica*, *127*(2), 145–152.

Snaith, R. P. (1996). Present use of the Hamilton Depression Rating Scale: Observation on method of assessment in research of depressive disorders. *British Journal of Psychiatry*, *168*(5), 594–597.

Solomon, D. A., Leon, A. C., Maser, J. D., et al. (2006). Distinguishing bipolar major depression from unipolar major depression with the Screening Assessment of Depression-Polarity (SAD-P). *Journal of Clinical Psychiatry*, *67*(3), 434–442.

Spearing, M. K., Post, R. M., Leverich, G. S., et al. (1997). Modification of the Clinical Global Impressions (CGI) Scale for use in bipolar illness (BP): The CGI-BP. *Psychiatry Research*, *73*(3), 159–171.

Spitzer, R. L., & Endicott, J. (1978). *Schedule for affective disorders and schizophrenia-change version* (3rd ed.). New York: New York State Psychiatric Institute, Biometrics Research.

Subero, M. M., Berk, L., Dodd, S., et al. (2013). To a broader concept of remission: Rating the health-related quality of life in bipolar disorder. *Journal of Affective Disorders*, *150*(2), 673–676.

Suppes, T., Vieta, E., Liu, S., et al. (2009). Maintenance treatment for patients with bipolar I disorder: Results from a North American study of quetiapine in combination with lithium or divalproex (trial 127). *American Journal of Psychiatry*, *166*(4), 476–488.

Swann, A. C., Secunda, S. K., Katz, M. M., et al. (1986). Lithium treatment of mania: Clinical characteristics, specificity of symptom change, and outcome. *Psychiatry Research*, *18*(2), 127–141.

Thalbourne, M. A., & Bassett, D. L. (1998). The Manic Depressiveness Scale: A preliminary effort at replication and extension. *Psychological Reports*, *83*(1), 75–80.

Thalbourne, M. A., Delin, P. S., & Bassett, D. L. (1994). An attempt to construct short scales measuring manic-depressive-like experience and behaviour. *British Journal of Clinical Psychology*, *33*(Pt 2), 205–207.

Thompson, P. M., Gonzalez, J. M., Singh, V., et al. (2010). Principal domains of behavioral psychopathology identified by the Bipolar Inventory of Signs and Symptoms Scale (BISS). *Psychiatry Research*, *175*(3), 221–226.

Tohen, M., Calabrese, J. R., Sachs. (2006). Randomized, placebo-controlled trial of olanzapine as maintenance therapy in patients with bipolar I disorder responding to acute treatment with olanzapine. *American Journal of Psychiatry, 163*(2), 247–256.

Tohen, M., Frank, E., Bowden, C. L., et al. (2009). The International Society for Bipolar Disorders (ISBD) task force report on the nomenclature of course and outcome in bipolar disorders. *Bipolar Disorders, 11*(5), 453–473.

Tohen, M., McDonnell, D. P., Case, M., et al. (2012). Randomised, double-blind, placebocontrolled study of olanzapine in patients with bipolar I depression. *British Journal of Psychiatry, 201*(5), 376–382.

Tohen, M., Zarate, C. A., Jr., Hennen, J., et al. (2003). The McLean-Harvard First-Episode Mania Study: Prediction of recovery and first recurrence. *American Journal of Psychiatry, 160*(12), 2099–2107.

Trivedi, M. H., Rush, A. J., Ibrahim, H. M., et al. (2004). The Inventory of Depressive Symptomatology, Clinician Rating (IDS-C) and Self-Report (IDS-SR), and the Quick Inventory of Depressive Symptomatology, Clinician Rating (QIDS-C) and Self-Report (QIDS-SR) in public sector patients with mood disorders: A psychometric evaluation. *Psychological Medicine, 34*(1), 73–82.

Trompenaars, F. J., Masthoff, E. D., Van Heck, G. L., et al. (2005). Content validity, construct validity, and reliability of the WHOQOL-Bref in a population of Dutch adult psychiatric outpatients. *Quality of Life Research, 14*(1), 151–160.

Unutzer, J., Simon, G., Pabiniak, C., et al. (1998). The treated prevalence of bipolar disorder in a large staff-model HMO. *Psychiatric Services (Washington, D.C.), 49*(8), 1072–1078.

van der Voort, T. Y., van Meijel, B., Goossens, P. J., et al. (2011). Collaborative care for patients with bipolar disorder: A randomised controlled trial. *BMC Psychiatry, 11*, 133.

Vieta, E., Suppes, T., Eggens, I., et al. (2008). Efficacy and safety of quetiapine in combination with lithium or divalproex for maintenance of patients with bipolar I disorder (international trial 126). *Journal of Affective Disorders, 109*(3), 251–263.

Washburn, J. J., West, A. E., & Heil, J. A. (2011). Treatment of pediatric bipolar disorder: A review. *Minerva Psichiatrica, 52*(1), 21–35.

Weisler, R. H., Calabrese, J. R., Thase, M. E., et al. (2008). Efficacy of quetiapine monotherapy for the treatment of depressive episodes in bipolar I disorder: A post hoc analysis of combined results from 2 double-blind, randomized, placebo-controlled studies. *Journal of Clinical Psychiatry, 69*(5), 769–782.

Weisler, R. H., Nolen, W. A., Neijber, A., et al. (2011). Continuation of quetiapine versus switching to placebo or lithium for maintenance treatment of bipolar I disorder (Trial 144: A randomized controlled study). *Journal of Clinical Psychiatry, 72*(11), 1452–1464.

Yatham, L. N., Fountoulakis, K. N., Rahman, Z., et al. (2013). Efficacy of aripiprazole versus placebo as adjuncts to lithium or valproate in relapse prevention of manic or mixed episodes in bipolar I patients stratified by index manic or mixed episode. *Journal of Affective Disorders, 147*(1–3), 365–372.

Young, A. H., McElroy, S. L., Bauer, M., et al. (2010a). A double-blind, placebo-controlled study of quetiapine and lithium monotherapy in adults in the acute phase of bipolar depression (EMBOLDEN I). *Journal of Clinical Psychiatry, 71*(2), 150–162.

Young, R. C., Biggs, J. T., Ziegler, V. E., et al. (1978). A rating scale for mania: Reliability, validity and sensitivity. *British Journal of Psychiatry, 133*, 429–435.

Young, R. C., Peasley-Miklus, C., & Shulberg, H. C. (2007). Mood ratings scales and the psychopathology of mania in old age: Selected applications and findings. In M. Sajatovic & F. Blow (Eds.), *Bipolar disorders in later life*. Baltimore, MD: Johns Hopkins Press.

Young, R. C., Schulberg, H. C., Gildengers, A. G., et al. (2010b). Conceptual and methodological issues in designing a randomized, controlled treatment trial for geriatric bipolar disorder: GERI-BD. *Bipolar Disorders, 12*(1), 56–67.

Youngstrom, E. A., Danielson, C. K., Findling, R. L., et al. (2002). Factor structure of the Young Mania Rating Scale for use with youths ages 5 to 17 years. *Journal of Clinical Child and Adolescent Psychology, 31*(4), 567–572.

Youngstrom, E. A., Findling, R. L., Danielson, C. K., et al. (2001). Discriminative validity of parent report of hypomanic and depressive symptoms on the General Behavior Inventory. *Psychological Assessment, 13*(2), 267–276.

Youngstrom, E. A., Findling, R. L., Youngstrom, J. K., et al. (2005). Toward an evidence-based assessment of pediatric bipolar disorder. *Journal of Clinical Child and Adolescent Psychology, 34*(3), 433–448.

Youngstrom, E. A., Frazier, T. W., Demeter, C., et al. (2008). Developing a 10-item mania scale from the Parent General Behavior inventory for children and adolescents. *Journal of Clinical Psychiatry, 69*(5), 831–839.

Zealley, A. K., & Aitken, R. C. (1969). Measurement of mood. *Proceedings of the Royal Society of Medicine, 62*(10), 993–996.

Chapter Ten

Clinical Applicability of Results from Drug Trials in Bipolar Disorder – An Attempt to Shed Light on a Complex Issue

Rasmus Wentzer Licht
Aalborg University Hospital, Aalborg, Denmark

CHAPTER OUTLINE

Clinical Trial Design Challenges in Mood Disorders. DOI: http://dx.doi.org/10.1016/B978-0-12-405170-6.00010-5

INTRODUCING THE PROBLEM

In all phases of bipolar disorder, psychopharmacologic treatment plays an important role, and, even though there are several relevant psychotropics available, better alternatives are needed and we need a better understanding of how to optimize the use of the existing agents (Grunze *et al.*, 2009, 2010, 2013). In the process of developing and improving our treatment options, the use of randomized clinical trials (RCTs) is crucial (Grof *et al.*, 1993). In principle and ideally, RCTs control for all other influences on outcome than the drug effect per se, and as such, the method is simple. However, designing and executing RCTs are complex and challenging processes, and the interpretation of the study results is equally complex and challenging (Cipriani & Geddes, 2009). Obviously, valid interpretations of the extent to which results from RCTs can be applied to certain specific clinical populations and clinical situations are essential for evidence-based medicine, which, at least in part, focuses on the match between the results of RCTs and the individual patients presenting in clinical practice (Geddes & Carney, 2009). Such interpretations are also essential, when guidance to clinicians is provided through the development of evidence-based treatment guidelines (Grunze *et al.*, 2009, 2010, 2013).

It can be argued that there are some specific issues within the field of psychiatry, and in particular within the field of bipolar disorder, in obtaining clinically applicable results from RCTs, issues that relate, for example, to difficulties in recruiting the most severely ill patients for study participation or to the very frequent occurrence of psychiatric comorbidity among bipolar patients (Vaidyanathan, Patrick & Iacono, 2012).

For various reasons, it is not always clear how to translate results from existing RCTs into clinical practice or whether they should be adopted at all, and, unfortunately, many trial reports do not explicitly address this issue. In addition, there are important clinical situations for which no or only a limited set of results can be applied (e.g., the frequent situation when a first-step treatment fails) (Grunze *et al.*, 2009). In such situations, the clinicians need to practice without strong guidance from evidence.

In the late 1990s, the issues outlined here above were phrased as the so-called gap between clinical research and clinical practice (Geddes & Harrison, 1997). This was around the time when the pharmaceutical industry began to see bipolar disorder as an upcoming market, and thereby began to move the field ahead, in particular by establishing valproate (Bowden *et al.*, 1994) and olanzapine (Tohen *et al.*, 1999) in mania through innovative, large RCTs, as alternatives to the standard treatment with typical antipsychotics (Licht, 1998).

Since then, most RCTs within the field of bipolar disorder have been driven by the pharmaceutical industry. This raises the question, to what extent these trials, which primarily aim at drug approval and/or promoting, have been able to meet the clinicians' needs.

AIMS AND METHODS

The aims of this chapter were three-fold. First, to address the issue of applicability of results from RCTs on drugs in bipolar disorder, in order to clarify this complex issue; this will include some considerations that are not specifically linked to bipolar disorder. Second, to address the question to what extent pharmaceutical industry-driven trials leading to regulatory drug approval in bipolar disorder provide results that are useful for clinical practice. Third, to discuss how clinicians potentially can and do develop pharmacotherapeutic strategies to overcome the potential limitations in the clinical applicability of results from bipolar drug trials.

The focus here was the clinical applicability of results from RCTs regarding the therapeutic effects of drugs, implying that the applicability of results regarding adverse effects will only be briefly addressed.

In addition, the focus of this chapter was RCTs in bipolar disorder evaluating drug effects in the population of nonelderly adults. However, a few notes will be given on generalizability of trial results across ages.

Due to the aims set up here, the chosen approach was essayistic, with the content based on the author's own work and reflections, common theory, and a relatively comprehensive selection of the literature, covering the major drug trials in acute mania, acute bipolar depression, and the maintenance phase of bipolar disorder. The trials to be discussed will mainly be pharmaceutically sponsored trials conducted with the purpose of regulatory drug approval, and, to a smaller extent, investigator-driven trials. Trials explicitly discussed will be cited directly, whereas trials discussed on a general level will be indirectly cited through other inclusive references (e.g., through references to treatment guidelines).

One way to evaluate empirically to what extent a given set of results from a conclusive RCT is actually applicable to patients treated in clinical practice, in the sense that an outcome similar to the one seen in the trial's patients can be obtained in a target population, might be to compare success rates in patients allocated to active treatment arms of the RCT with those rates obtained under routine conditions as demonstrated in an observational study. However, such comparisons are influenced by selection bias and will not be addressed here. Likewise, the pharmacoepidemiologic literature describing which treatments are actually applied in clinical practice will not be addressed since many other factors other than the clinical applicability of trials results determine the behavior of clinicians. To this end, it should be noted, that the clinical applicability of trial results as defined in the following section is considered to be a matter of qualitative statement indicating a level of recommendation based on scientific and clinical reasoning and judgment, and it should be clearly differentiated from an actual application of such results and in particular from the actual application of a treatment per se.

CONCEPTUAL FRAMEWORK
Unfolding the Basic Concepts

Of high relevance for the following, three interrelated concepts need to be defined and disentangled, that is, internal validity, external validity, and clinical applicability. Besides being used in clinical epidemiology, the terms internal and external validity are also used in psychometric theory (Bech, 1995), but this is not relevant here. In the present context, internal validity refers to the credibility of the comparison (e.g., drug versus placebo) per se, that is, the extent to which systematic errors (or biases) are avoided (Rothman, 1986). The advantage of performing randomization is that selection bias is thereby avoided. In contrast, external validity refers to the generalizability of the comparison, that is, to the extent to which specific statements about the comparison can be transferred to specific subjects under specific circumstances (Schene, Wijngaarden & Baaren-Marcelis, 1994). Sometimes the term selection bias is used to describe a selection prior to randomization; such selection should more correctly be considered as a factor impacting generalizability (Rothman, 1986). Two important points should be stressed here. First, the generalizability is not solely confined by the representativeness of the study subjects; it is also confined by the pre-randomization study conditions, that is, the procedures that the study subjects underwent before randomization. In maintenance studies, a specific study condition could, for example, be the requirement that patients should have demonstrated an acute response to the treatment in question before randomization. Second, internal validity is a prerequisite for generalizability; if the comparison in question is completely biased, there is nothing to be generalized, no matter how much the randomized patients are representative of a certain clinical population (Rothman, 1986). In addition, generalizability requires that the study is well powered. On top of the concepts of internal validity and generalizability, there is the concept of clinical applicability. Literally, the concept may seem identical with the concept of generalizability, but in the author's interpretation, it has a slightly different meaning, which relates to the perspective. Where internal validity and generalizability are concepts closely linked to the RCT in question, the concept of clinical applicability is linked to the clinical situation. The former concepts cover the validity of the specific trial results per se, whereas the latter concept covers the perspective of the evidence-oriented clinician who asks which results can be used in the management of a specific clinical problem. If no results matching the clinical problem can be found, the task for the clinician is to find results matching as much as possible even though this implies that the treatment decision may transcend the strict generalizability of the results. Examples of such decision-making could be:

1. a manic patient with comorbid alcohol abuse is treated with valproate even though this has not been formally tested in an RCT since patients with

comorbid alcohol abuse were excluded from major RCTs demonstrating efficacy of valproate in mania (Bowden *et al.*, 1994);

2. a bipolar depressed severely suicidal patient is treated with quetiapine even though patients with suicidal ideation were excluded from the trials demonstrating efficacy of quetiapine in bipolar depression (Calabrese *et al.*, 2005; Thase *et al.*, 2006);

3. a patient with bipolar disorder, type II with recurrent depression is treated prophylactically with lamotrigine even though such a property is only documented in patients with bipolar disorder, type I (Calabrese *et al.*, 2003).

As illustrated by the examples above, on the one hand the concept of clinical applicability of results from RCTs may be broader than the concept of generalizability but on the other hand, through its inherent clinical perspective, the former concept is a bit narrower than the latter, since not only the pre-randomization study conditions but also the post-randomization study conditions and procedures must be relevant and applicable to a routine clinical setting. In addition, even though trial results on a specific drug may be highly generalizable, the clinical applicability of these results may be reduced due to tolerability and safety concerns from the clinicians' and patients' perspective. Taken together, the concept of clinical applicability focuses on the needs of the clinician and ultimately of those of the patient. By focusing on the extent to which trial results relevantly can be applied to specific clinical situations, the concept indirectly points at the clinical situations that are not covered by results from RCTs. Thereby, the aim of the RCT (e.g., drug approval or improved management of insufficient treatment response to first-step treatment) is raised as a major point of interest.

A note of clinical importance should be made even though it may seem trivial: the applicability of results from RCTs should be evaluated not only when they are positive, but indeed also when they are negative, so the border between negative evidence and lack of evidence becomes clear.

The full clinical applicability of results from a specific RCT obviously cannot be evaluated until after the execution of the trial since there will be influences from, for example, the dropout rates and the collected study sample. However, some important aspects of the potential clinical applicability of the study can be addressed a priori on the basis of the study design and the study goal.

Selection of Subjects to Randomized Clinical Trials

When planning an RCT, the starting point is the target population, that is, the population to which the results ideally should be generalizable (e.g., manic inpatients in need of drug treatment), and formal inclusion criteria matching the target population, specifying such variables as age, diagnosis, and severity, are set up (Elwood, 1988). The study sample is drawn from the source population (e.g., admitted patients in various treatment settings, including manic patients) (Licht *et al.*, 1997). Patients identified in this way are potentially eligible for randomization since they represent the target population. The example with the manic patients is simple. Another, more complex, example is when the target population is stabilized bipolar patients in need of maintenance treatment (Weisler *et al.*, 2011). Here, the eligible patients are stabilized patients. If they are selected as remitting on and tolerating a specific drug, then this needs to be incorporated into the description of the target population.

Subsequently, the population of eligible patients is diminished due to necessary exclusion criteria set up for safety, ethical, and/or other reasons. In many trial reports, the inclusion and exclusion criteria are simply coalesced as selection criteria. This approach reflects that if patients during screening are meeting an exclusion criterion they are most often not assessed for the fulfilment of inclusion criteria. Moreover, for some factors, it can be questioned whether they should lead to an inclusion or to an exclusion criterion; substance abuse for example can in its absence be considered an inclusion criterion or in its presence an exclusion criterion. The advantage of separating the two types of criteria and assessing patients for fulfilment of inclusion criteria prior to assessing whether they meet exclusion criteria is that it makes it possible to examine the exact disposition of the eligible patients regarding selection factors in order to estimate the generalizability of study results in more details (e.g., whether consenting and nonconsenting patients differ beyond their attitude to the trial). Unfortunately, very few such attempts have been reported within the field of bipolar disorder (Bowden *et al.*, 1995; Greil *et al.*, 1993; Licht *et al.*, 1997). One main reason for this is the workload it takes to carefully assess and record a number of patients much higher than the number required for the conduct of the trial as such. Another good reason is that the source population may be selected anyway, as discussed in the paragraph below.

Ideally, to ensure generalizability and replicability of the study findings, the eligible patients must be a random sample of the target population (Rothman, 1986). The prerequisite for this is that the source population comprises subjects that are fully representative of the target population. If the source population, for example, is patients referred to a facility for treatment-resistant patients, such representativeness is most likely not the case. In fact, to be fully representative to typical patients presenting in ordinary, not specialized treatment settings, the source population needs to come from a well-defined geographical catchment area. Unfortunately, only a few countries (e.g., Denmark) have an organization of health care that allows such recruitment (Licht *et al.*, 1997). To be a random sample, the eligible patients should also be identified through screening of consecutively presenting patients (e.g., consecutively admitted patients), since otherwise, the selection may be influenced by unknown or informal selection criteria with the result that the study sample is not identified solely by the formal selection criteria. Attempts to characterize the actual patient flow from screening to randomization above may reduce the informal selection of patients. Taken together, the less the study sample can be considered a random sample of the target population, the more uncertain the generalizability of the trial results will be.

Narrow Versus Broad Generalizability

There are two dimensions that can be formulated as dichotomies regarding generalizability of specific trial results (i.e., the dichotomy of respectively unknown/uncertain versus known/specified generalizability and broad versus narrow generalizability). The latter dimension obviously calls for specification if possible. As mentioned above, an informal selection, for example, of mildly ill patients, leads to an unknown/uncertain generalizability. This may be the case in complex multicenter trials, where each center is supposed to recruit only a limited number of patients. As to the second dichotomy, in explanatory (efficacy) trials aiming at optimizing the likelihood of finding a signal if it is there, relatively homogenous study samples, characterized by patients without comorbidities and with a high degree of cooperativeness due to the requirement of many assessments, are usually selected, making the generalizability relatively narrow (Sackett, 2011). In contrast, in pragmatic (effectiveness) trials, a relatively broad generalizability is usually obtained through the use of a minimum of exclusion criteria and attempts to achieve relatively high consent rates by applying simple study procedures (Sackett, 2011). The broadening of generalizability in the latter type of trials is generally associated with lower chances of detecting potential group differences due to high dropout rates, low compliance, or inclusion of nonresponding subgroups. Even when a high internal validity can be obtained in these trials, the potential inclusion of nonresponding subgroups will reduce the potential overall effect sizes, if they can be detected at all despite their presence due to the corresponding higher requirements to the sample size. However, the border between these two prototypes of trials is not clear, and some trials are in between the two (Geddes, 2005).

Effect Size and Clinical Applicability of Trial Results

The translation of trial results into clinical practice may also depend on the effect size and how this is reported. Since all results from RCTs are group effects, it is never possible to know whether a given patient will respond to a given treatment no matter how valid and accurate the estimate of effect size is. However, the higher the effect size (statistically significantly different from zero) is, in terms of a categorically defined between-group treatment effect, and thereby the lower number needed to treat (Cook & Sackett, 1995), the higher is the clinician's possibility of predicting a treatment response in an individual patient, since the effect size as a between-group difference in proportions simply equals the likelihood of response in an individual patient caused by the treatment in question. Moreover, from the patient's perspective, the higher the likelihood of effect, the more real and less theoretical will the communicated trial results appear. Drawing the likelihood of a response in an individual into focus when discussing the applicability of trial results underscores the importance of providing effect sizes as categorically measures in trial reports.

As outlined above, the likelihood of an added benefit from a specific treatment in an individual patient may be related to the wideness of generalizability, since a broadening of generalizability is often associated with smaller effect sizes while a narrowing is often associated with larger effect sizes.

Generalizability Across Classification Systems

Generalizing trial results from patients fulfilling specific diagnostic criteria according to one classification system (e.g., the Diagnostic and Statistical Manual of Mental Disorders, Fourth Edition (DSM-IV) (American Psychiatric Association, 2004) to patients meeting criteria for the same diagnosis but according to another classification system (e.g., International Classification of Diseases (ICD)-10 (World Health Organization, 1992), might create a problem, since the diagnosis obviously is the major inclusion criteria across all RCTs. Likewise, changes from earlier to later versions of a classification system (e.g., from DSM-IV to Diagnostic and Statistical Manual of Mental Disorders, Fifth Edition (DSM-5) (American Psychiatric Association, 2013)), might influence generalizability of trial results. However, regarding the DSM-IV versus the ICD-10, the differences in the criteria for mania, defining the core feature of bipolar disorder, are without importance (Licht, Bysted & Christensen, 2001). Also regarding Diagnostic and Statistical Manual of Mental Disorders, Third Edition (DSM-III) (American Psychiatric Association, 1980) and subsequent versions, the criteria for mania are similar.

As to the major trials addressing the treatment of mania, all of these, with a few exceptions (Bowden *et al.*, 1994; Prien, Caffey & Klett, 1972), have been conducted in the era of DSM-IV. The most recent transition from DSM-IV to DSM-5, the latter defining mania more restrictively than the former by adding a requirement of increased activity to the primary criterion, presumably will not have any influence on the generalizability of results from the available major RCTs on mania, since most trial patients fulfilling the entry requirement of a certain degree of severity of mania most likely will also have increased activity at some level.

Regarding maintenance trials, the major challenge is that some earlier trials do not separate bipolar disorder type I and type II (Goodwin & Jamison, 1990). Since the most important maintenance trials are conducted on bipolar disorder type I patients, it should also be noted that the ICD-10 does not separate explicitly the two subtypes of bipolar disorder.

For bipolar depression, again, there are only subtle differences between the DSM-IV, in which era the major RCTs have been conducted, and the ICD-10, and the criteria are unchanged from DSM-IV to DSM-5.

Concerning mixed states, the situation is more complex. In most trials enrolling patients with mixed states, these patients are diagnosed according to DSM-IV, implying that the results cannot necessarily be generalized to patients with a mixed state according to the ICD-10, where this state is much more loosely defined and also covers patients with depression and a few concurrent manic symptoms. This caution also applies to the generalizability of results to patients with the mixed feature specifier in the DSM-5.

Generalizability Across Age

Regarding age, all RCTs define an age range as an important inclusion criterion. The study population is most often restricted to be nonelderly adults, for example, subjects from 18 to 65 years of age. Three main reasons for this, relating to safety, ethics, feasibility, and success, can be identified. Conducting trials in children/adolescents and in the very elderly obviously may carry a relatively large risk of safety issues. In the elderly population, the risk of adverse drug effects simply may be higher due to risk factors such as somatic comorbid conditions, and in the younger, adverse effects such as weight gain may be a more crucial. In addition, in both groups, there are special concerns regarding informed consent. Likewise, and related to the former reasons, recruitment of younger and elderly patients may be difficult; the more atypical clinical presentation of bipolar disorder in the younger population also may add to recruitment difficulties. Finally, the likelihood of getting a positive outcome of a trial may be relatively low in the extreme age groups due to potentially higher dropout rates, due to a more dubious compliance and potentially due to biologic factors. As to the latter point, results from RCTs on antidepressants in younger patients with unipolar depression indicate a relatively low efficacy of antidepressants, in particular of tricyclic antidepressants (Tsapakis *et al.*, 2008), and in the elderly there seems to be a higher risk of organic bipolar disorder, eventually leading to treatment resistance (Mendez, 2000).

Although trial results from the nonelderly adults cannot necessarily be applied to the other age groups, the clinician may need to apply such results, when younger or older patients come into clinical situations that require intervention with drugs. An example of such common practice is the continuation of a successful lithium treatment even though the patient ages beyond the inclusion criteria of age in maintenance trials. Fortunately, the evidence on treatment options in young people with bipolar disorder is growing, in particular regarding the treatment of mania (Goldstein, Sassi & Diler, 2012). Interestingly, the only trial conducted in patients with bipolar disorder and comorbid substance abuse is conducted in adolescents (Geller *et al.*, 1998). It is remarkable, that no trial on mania in older people has yet been published. However, one trial is hopefully on its way (Young *et al.*, 2010b).

As an additional note, it should be pointed out that the age range from 18 to 65 years in itself covers heterogeneous study populations of patients in term of not only age but also in terms of age of onset of illness.

Generalizability Across Drugs

The general and straightforward answer to the question whether it is possible to generalize results based on an RCT on one drug to patients treated with another drug is negative. The situation is more complex when considering drugs within the same class. However, at this point, a distinction between various classes of drugs should be performed. It is beyond any doubt that the antimanic effect of valproate in mania cannot be seen as a class effect, since there are examples of anticonvulsants with clearly no effect on mania (Grunze *et al.*, 2009). In contrast, for antipsychotics (i.e., drugs that to some extent block the dopamine D-2 receptors), the hypothesis that an antimanic effect is a class effect linked to this blocking property has never been rejected (Berk *et al.*, 2007). A third class of drugs giving rise to a still ongoing controversy within the field is the class of antidepressants; besides the discussion of their efficacy and safety, there is a discussion of a potential class effect (Pacchiarotti *et al.*, 2013).

Generalizability and Adverse Effects

Generalizability of results on adverse effects as such follows the same basic principles as generalizability of results on therapeutic effects. However, it should be emphasized that the generalizability and applicability of results on adverse effects on the one hand may be broader than that of results on therapeutic effects in the sense that such results may be applied across diagnosis and treatment phases. On the other hand, it may be narrower when it comes to application of results from groups of nonelderly adults to younger and elderly groups.

Another aspect of adverse effects to be addressed in this context is the impact of such effects on the applicability of results on therapeutic effects from RCTs. Obviously, to be applicable into clinical practice trial results should indicate a favorable side effect profile of the drug in question. In addition, general safety concerns play a role even though not particularly addressed in the specific trial. It may for example not be justifiable to use tamoxifen, an antiestrogen, into routine practice for the treatment of mania, even though there are positive widely generalizable trial results available (Yildiz *et al.*, 2008). Another example is the actual replacement of typical antipsychotics with atypical antipsychotics in the treatment of mania since the mid-1990s (Larsen *et al.*, 2009; Licht *et al.*, 1994), which may reflect that the relatively low risk of neurologic side effects of the atypical antipsychotics potentially have contributed to a relatively high degree of clinical applicability of the trial results on these agents.

INDUSTRY-DRIVEN VERSUS INVESTIGATOR-DRIVEN TRIALS IN GENERAL

The industry-driven RCTs are initiated, designed, and sponsored by a pharmaceutical company. These trials are generally conducted with the primary purpose of obtaining regulatory approval (phase III trials) or with the purpose of postmarketing promotion (phase IV trials). Typically, the approval trials are placebo-controlled trials belonging to the former mentioned category of explanatory efficacy trials, designed to maximize the sensitivity of signal detecting with a corresponding relatively narrow generalizability of study results. The postmarketing trials are generally comparative, and the patients recruited to these trials are often more representative of patients seen in clinical practice than patients recruited to placebo-controlled trials. However, these trials may experience various sources of bias (e.g., due to improper dose regimen regarding the drug from the competitor) (Vieta & Cruz, 2012).

Investigator-driven RCTs are designed and conducted by the investigators themselves and funded through unrestricted grants. These trials are often comparative, and with their pragmatic approach, they generally include more representative patients, but the drawback is a reduction in the signal-to-noise ratio, which in combination with low study power may lead to negative results. These trials are also often open, which may bias the comparison and thereby limit what can actually be generalized.

The border between industry-driven and investigator-driven trials is far from clear. Many of industry-driven trials are designed and executed through assistance from experts within the field, and these experts may also assist with writing up the final report, and the grants for the latter trials may be provided by pharmaceutical companies. In between the two types of trials, there are investigator-initiated trials, where the idea comes from the independent investigator(s), but with the study being developed in collaboration between the investigator(s) and the company and being fully or partly sponsored by the drug company.

GENERALIZABILITY AND CLINICAL APPLICABILITY OF TRIAL RESULTS IN BIPOLAR DISORDER
Mania

Until the pharmaceutical industry started focusing on mania in the 1990s (Bowden *et al.*, 1994; Tohen *et al.*, 1999), the RCTs were essentially investigator-driven (Licht, 1998). However, even though the patients in these earlier trials may have been relatively broadly selected, the clinical applicability of the results is limited by the fact that the trials, with a few exceptions (Prien *et al.*, 1972), were underpowered (Licht, 1998); also in most of the trials, no specific mania rating scale was applied.

The large study samples in the huge number of modern approval trials in mania are highly selected. Besides being selected through formal selection criteria (Storosum *et al.*, 2004), there is a risk of unknown (and unreported) informal selection since only a minor (and not random) proportion of potentially eligible patients may be approached (Licht, 2001). In addition, many of the participating centers may be tertiary centers recruiting relatively treatment-refractory patients.

Considering the large number of positive trials, the vast majority being approval trials, the drug–placebo differences are remarkably consistent across the trials, with pooled responder rates of 48% and 31%, respectively in drug and placebo groups (Yildiz *et al.*, 2011), with response defined as a 50% reduction or more on a relevant mania rating scale over 3 weeks. Compatible with this, with the exception of two trials (Niufan *et al.*, 2008; Prien *et al.*, 1972), no comparative trials in mania have demonstrated any clinically significant differences between any of the drugs proven to work in mania (Grunze *et al.*, 2009).

Even though lithium has been found to be equally effective to quetiapine and valproate (Bowden *et al.*, 1994, 2005, 2010), it was inferior to chlorpromazine (Prien *et al.*, 1972) and olanzapine (Niufan *et al.*, 2008). In the former of these trials, which was investigator-driven, chlorpromazine was superior to lithium in highly active manic patients, whereas in mildly active manic patients, lithium and chlorpromazine were comparable. The comparative trials mentioned above comprised three-arm approval trials with an active control besides the placebo arm, postmarketing noninferiority trials, and superiority trials.

In all the approval trials on mania, the study samples seem to be selected in somewhat similar ways by excluding the most severely and/or uncooperative manic patients and patients who had various comorbid conditions including substance abuse. This indicates that the generalizability of the trial results generally seems to be narrowed in the same way across all the drugs tested to be positive. However, part of the results of the study by Prien *et al.* (1972) (i.e., the part indicating inferiority of lithium, cited above can be specifically generalized to highly active manic patients), reflected in some guidelines recommending lithium only in mildly active patients (American Psychiatric Association, 2002). In such a recommendation, it is assumed that the results of inferiority of lithium compared with chlorpromazine in highly active patients in fact can be generalized to lithium compared with other antipsychotics as well, which seems reasonable. Regarding other potential differential generalizabilities of trial results due to differential findings in clinical subgroups of manic patients, all the trials included up to 50% psychotic patients who, across all drugs including lithium, seem to respond to the same degree as the nonpsychotic patients (Grunze *et al.*, 2009; Licht, 2006). Importantly, this broadens the generalizability of the results from all trials, again in the same direction across all drugs. Interestingly, a post-hoc analysis of data from an RCT indicated a slightly differential generalizability of results due to slightly differential effect on various symptom profiles of valproate and lithium in various clinical subgroups (Swann *et al.*, 2002).

As to the generalizability of the results from the major lithium trials, it should be noted that it is further specified by the pre-randomization study conditions, that is, to patients that agree on the mandatory serum lithium monitoring.

In line with the fact that manic patients in trials are highly selected as outlined above, it is often claimed that results from these trials cannot be applied to the most severely ill manic patients. However, there are data indicating that the placebo response decreases with increasing severity of mania (Bowden *et al.*, 2006), implying that the effect size in fact will increase in more severely ill patients, given of course that the drug in question has an antimanic effect. Likewise, Pope *et al.* (1991), recruiting their study sample from two hospitals by screening manic patients admitted consecutively, obtained a considerably larger valproate–placebo effect size than that obtained in the multicenter trial by Bowden *et al.* (1994), explained by a much lower placebo response rate in the former trial. Presumably, patients in the investigator-driven study by Pope *et al.* (1991) were more severely ill than patients in the approval study by Bowden *et al.* (1994) due to the different recruitment procedures.

One of the most important issues in the management of mania is how to move beyond first-step treatment. Given the fact that at least 50% of manic patients in RCTs will not respond to any first-step treatment after 3–4 weeks (Grunze et al., 2009), the evidence addressing second-step treatment is highly insufficient. In approval trials, patients not responding to a first-step treatment are generally not excluded, but no subgroup analyses potentially providing results applicable to this clinical situation are available. A number of approval trials have evaluated the addition of an antipsychotic as compared with placebo on top of a mood stabilizer in patients insufficiently responding to the mood-stabilizer alone (Smith et al., 2007). However, the study conditions prior to randomization are not clearly described in any of these trials. Some patients are included because of insufficient prophylactic response and some patients are included due to insufficient acute response to the mood stabilizer, after varying periods of time, and the exact distribution of these conditions is generally not reported. Accordingly, the generalizability regarding efficacy is uncertain, reflecting what is often neglected when these trial results are interpreted, namely that they essentially were conducted to demonstrate the safety of the combination of an atypical antipsychotic with a mood stabilizer as an additional requirement for drug approval. Only one RCT, which was investigator-initiated but industry sponsored, addressed directly the management of patients insufficiently responding to first-step treatment. Unfortunately, this trial was never completed (Licht & Bech, 2009). In addition, drug combinations from start of treatment have been properly evaluated in only one (investigator-driven) RCT (Muller-Oerlinghausen et al., 2000). This trial is the major evidence behind the treatment guideline recommendation that a combination of valproate and an atypical antipsychotic should be considered in severe mania (American Psychiatric Association, 2002), since it is the only trial in which the combination is compared with an antipsychotic alone. This recommendation reasonably goes beyond the generalizability of the trial results per se; even though the trial was conducted on hospitalized patients, the most severely manic patients presumably were not enrolled. In addition, the findings are generalized to atypical antipsychotics in general, while the trial in fact examined the typical antipsychotic perphenazine. The lack of trials covering the management of treatment-resistant manic patients has led to the occasional application of trial results on clozapine in schizophrenia (Nielsen, Kane & Correll, 2012).

The management of mania appearing in a patient receiving a maintenance treatment is partly, but only partly, covered by the trials evaluating the addition of an atypical antipsychotic in addition to a mood-stabilizer (Smith et al., 2007).

Bipolar Depression

The largest issue with bipolar depression is not limitation of generalizability of trial results, but the limitation of number of trials addressing the various treatment options in bipolar depression (Grunze et al., 2010). The drug with the highest degree of evidence for efficacy in bipolar depression is quetiapine (Grunze et al., 2010). Until very recently, when lurasidone obtained regulatory approval (pivotal studies yet unpublished), quetiapine was the only drug with monotherapy approval for this indication. In the pivotal placebo-controlled trials of quetiapine demonstrating relatively large drug–placebo effect sizes, suicidal patients were excluded. Likewise, severely depressed patients, unable to provide informed consent or requiring electroconvulsive therapy, were not enrolled. Interestingly, randomization of bipolar depressed patients with psychotic symptoms was allowed (Calabrese et al., 2005; Thase et al., 2006). However, no data were given in the reports on how many patients with psychotic features were actually enrolled in the trials. The author has made many attempts through contacting the sponsor to get this information, but it has not been possible. Here it should be borne in mind that even though the selection criteria of a trial reflect the target population (here depressed nonsuicidal bipolar patients with or without psychotic symptoms), the results can only be generalized to this target population if the randomized sample can be considered a random sample of this target population. Therefore, it is uncertain whether these trial results can be generalized to the population of depressed bipolar patients with psychotic symptoms, implying that, in a worst case scenario, the trial results can be generalized only to the population of bipolar depressed patients without psychotic symptoms, as is the general case in trials in bipolar depression; even for unipolar psychotic depression, the evidence base is extremely poor (Wijkstra, Schubart & Nolen, 2009). Another uncertainty about the generalizability of the results from these trials relates to the pre-randomization study conditions. In the reports, it was mentioned that patients on antidepressants had these drugs discontinued before randomization, but again it has not been possible to get any information on which proportion of the patients actually had an antidepressant discontinued. Discontinuation of an antidepressant may lead to a discontinuation syndrome (Schatzberg et al., 2006) or to worsening of depression in case a relative response to the antidepressant has taken place. These factors may have increased the drug–placebo signal in a subset of patients, since quetiapine quickly ameliorates anxiety and sleep problems, and thereby potentially may have contributed to the relatively large overall effect sizes.

Another approval trial of quetiapine included lithium as an internal control of assay sensitivity, but no statistically significant superiority of lithium over placebo was found (Young et al., 2010a), thereby questioning a number of earlier investigator-driven trials supporting the beneficial role of this drug in bipolar depression (Licht, 2012). However, lithium doses were relatively low, and the pre-randomization study conditions, similar to those discussed above, also may have contributed to the negative results and limited their generalizability.

Regarding lamotrigine, when the five negative approval studies were analyzed together, a drug–placebo signal was found (Geddes, Calabrese & Goodwin, 2009); the signal was larger and clinically relevant in the subgroup of more severely depressed patients. This meta-analysis indicates indirectly that the essentially negative results of each of the approval trials may only be generalized to populations of patients with a relatively mild degree of bipolar depression.

The use of antidepressants for bipolar depression is still one of the most debated issues within the field (Pacchiarotti *et al.*, 2013), and the controversy somewhat relates to the generalizability of results from RCTs. For various reasons, the number of conclusive placebo-controlled trials addressing the efficacy of these agents in bipolar depression is very low (Licht *et al.*, 2008). The closest we come to an approval trial on an antidepressant is the pivotal trial for the approval of the combination of fluoxetine and olanzapine for bipolar depression (Tohen *et al.*, 2003). Two questions can be raised regarding the generalizability of the results from this trial. First, can these results showing superiority of olanzapine plus fluoxetine over olanzapine plus placebo (and superiority over placebo alone) be considered a proof of the efficacy of fluoxetine as such and be generalized accordingly, or do they only relate to the combination as such versus monotherapy, assuming a specific synergistic effect inherent in the former? Second, can the results of fluoxetine and of the combination be generalized to other selective serotonin reuptake inhibitor antidepressants and other combinations of such antidepressants and atypical antipsychotics? Obviously, these questions cannot be properly answered. One of the main sources of evidence for no additional benefits of adding an antidepressant to a mood stabilizer is the RCT by Sachs *et al.* (2007) conducted within the framework of the Systematic Treatment Enhancement Program for Bipolar Disorder (STEP-BD). However, several points should be taken into account when generalizing these negative findings. First, there was a high rate of comorbid psychiatric conditions in the study sample. Second, at randomization, patients had already been treated within the STEP-BD for around 6 months on average, and presumably a substantial number of patients may have shown nonresponse to other antidepressants before randomization. Third, additional treatment with antipsychotics, some of them known to be somewhat effective in treating bipolar depression, was allowed, and a proportion of patients also participated in a trial on psychosocial intervention. Finally, the findings may only be confined to the actually tested antidepressants (i.e., bupropion and paroxetine). An additional aspect of generalizability that is related to the discussion of the use of antidepressants in bipolar depression is whether results from trials on unipolar depression can be generalized to patients with bipolar depression or to a subset of these (Moller, Grunze & Broich, 2006). Again, this question cannot be answered with our current level of knowledge.

Besides the trial cited above examining a combination of fluoxetine and olanzapine, one investigator-initiated trial supported the beneficial effect of adding lamotrigine to patients already on lithium (van der Loos *et al.*, 2009). Although a proportion of the patients in the latter trial presumably were experiencing a break-through-prophylaxis depression, the results of both trials may be applied to second-step treatment situations for bipolar depression, for which there is an absence of RCTs.

Mixed States

Despite the fact that a number of drugs have obtained approval on the indication of mixed state, no trial has been conducted solely for such an approval (Vieta, 2005). In all cases, the approval has been given on the basis of post-hoc analyses on subsets of patients, who, while being enrolled in the approval trials of mania, at the same time, fulfilled the criteria of a mixed state. Generally, this has been accomplished simply by allowing patients to have depressive symptoms concurrent with a full manic syndrome. What can be generalized from these trials is that patients with mixed state will have the same likelihood for an antimanic response as those patients with a nonmixed mania. Or more importantly, it cannot be generalized that patients with mixed state can expect an improvement in the core depressive symptoms due to the treatment in question. Even though it has been demonstrated in many of these trials that the treatment reduces the score on a depression scale, it should be remembered that many items on such scales are overlapping with items typically for mania, for example, sleep disturbances and agitation. The only drugs that have been demonstrated to be better than placebo regarding core depressive symptoms in mixed state is olanzapine in combination with lithium or valproate (Tohen *et al.*, 2002). Asenapine seemingly also has specific potentials regarding depressive symptoms in the context of mania (McIntyre & Wong, 2012).

The only large, conclusive trial that has primarily enrolled patients with mixed state was a postmarketing trial finding olanzapine plus valproate to be superior to olanzapine plus placebo (Houston *et al.*, 2009).

Ironically, one of the few atypical antipsychotics that has not been approved for the treatment of mixed state is quetiapine (Vieta, 2005). In the pivotal studies on mania, patients with depressive symptoms were excluded. Given the evidence for the efficacy of this drug in mania and in bipolar depression, the question is whether the combined results from the trials in mania and in bipolar depression could be applied to patients in a mixed state. This is an open question, and even though such applicability might seem reasonable, it should be remembered that depression occurring in the context of concurrent mania might be different to depression occurring separately in time from mania (Koukopoulos & Ghaemi, 2009).

Maintenance

With one exception (Bowden *et al.*, 2000), in all maintenance trials conducted for drug approval, the study samples have been enriched, that is, the patients have been required to demonstrate various degrees of acute phase response and/or tolerance to the drug in question prior to randomization (Grunze *et al.*, 2013). In addition, these trials are discontinuation trials, where the responding patients are randomly allocated to either continued treatment with the drug in question or to treatment with placebo (or an active comparator). Under such conditions, a high risk of early re-emerging of mood symptoms in the placebo (or active comparator) group may increase the likelihood of a signal in favor of the drug in question. Likewise, the likelihood of successful drug versus placebo prevention of later re-emerging of symptoms is maximized. The pre-randomization enriched study conditions obviously narrow the generalizability of the study results. However, it can be argued that the clinical applicability none-the-less is still broad, since such study conditions match a common clinical situation, that is, the continuing of a treatment that seemingly worked acutely. In contrast, it can be argued that it is more common that the clinician does not know which drug or combination of drugs actually made the patient respond if not time only, which in terms of applicability advocates for not selecting study patients on the basis of their acute response. In the approval trial that was not enriched, valproate was compared with placebo, with lithium added as a third arm for control of the assay sensitivity (Bowden et al., 2000). Since lithium (and valproate) did not perform better than placebo on the primary outcome measure, the trial can be considered a failed trial. The main reason for this is probably that the majority of the patients had a relatively low risk of recurrence (Bowden et al., 1995). However, in a post-hoc analysis of a subsample of patients who were treated successfully with valproate during mania prior to randomization, valproate was found to be superior to placebo (McElroy et al., 2008). The study conditions regarding this subsample resemble the enriched study conditions outlined above.

Some of the enriched, discontinuation approval trials introduced lithium (Bowden et al., 2003; Calabrese et al., 2003; Weisler et al., 2011), and one olanzapine (Vieta et al., 2012) in a nonenriched way as a comparator to control for the assay sensitivity, thereby broadening the generalizability of the specific findings regarding this third arm to euthymic patients that, for example, are untreated or have their acute treatment discontinued after remission. Despite this broadening, the effect size of lithium (or olanzapine) versus placebo was comparable to that of the drug investigated under enriched conditions. Here it should also be noted that the discontinuation effect affected this third arm in the same way as it affected the placebo arm. Most likely, results obtained under nonenriched conditions can be applied to clinical situations resembling enriched conditions. At least, there are no data rejecting this hypothesis.

The post-randomization discontinuation condition mimics the routine situation when patients stop the medication given acutely immediately after improvement has been obtained, for example, due to poor compliance after discharge, potentially related to side effects. However, even though results of a signal detection under this condition cover such abrupt drug discontinuation, it does not necessarily imply that the results cover whether a given drug prevents against true recurrences in the long term, that is, emerging symptoms independent of the acute episode (Frank et al., 1991). Attempts to overcome the interference of the discontinuation effect with the detection of a true preventive effect have been done in the field of unipolar disorder by interposing a drug-free period, but in more severely ill patients, such attempts are not clinically feasible (Licht, 2013). Another commonly used approach is to make additional outcome analyses excluding early treatment emergent episodes (Goodwin et al., 2004).

In the approval maintenance trials incorporating a lithium arm, inclusion of patients with prior nonresponse to lithium was allowed, which should be taken into account when the results regarding lithium are interpreted. In one head-to-head comparison of olanzapine against lithium, a substantial proportion of patients had in fact demonstrated prior insufficient response to lithium, increasing the likelihood of a signal in favor of olanzapine (Tohen *et al.*, 2005). Even though numbers are often small, subgroup analyses of patients with and without prior insufficient response to lithium would contribute to specify the generalizability of such trial results.

The generalizability of results from maintenance trials is also potentially influenced by the polarity of the index episode, since the index episode predicts the polarity of recurrence (Calabrese *et al.*, 2004). Illustrating this point, in the trial comparing quetiapine with placebo, where the patients had an index episode of depression, no mania preventive effect of quetiapine over placebo could be found (Young *et al.*, 2014), whereas such an effect was found in the other pivotal study including patients with either mania or depression (Weisler *et al.*, 2011). However, in the pivotal trials of lamotrigine (Bowden *et al.*, 2003; Calabrese *et al.*, 2003), covering both patients with an index episode of mania and patients with an index episode of depression, the response pattern was similar across the polarity of index episode.

Regarding the differential response patterns of various preventive drugs, for example, lamotrigine preventing depression better than preventing mania (Goodwin *et al.*, 2004), it is reasonably assumed that the benefit of certain drugs may be maximized by applying the corresponding trial results in accordance with the predominance of polarity of individual patients (Colom *et al.*, 2006).

Four recent investigator-driven maintenance RCTs have provided comparative results regarding lithium versus alternative mood stabilizers, obtained under conditions not favoring any of the comparators (Geddes *et al.*, 2010; Greil *et al.*, 1997; Hartong *et al.*, 2003; Licht *et al.*, 2010). These comparisons were characterized by not selecting the study samples based on acute response to any of the drugs under comparison and thereby also by avoiding skewed post-randomization drug discontinuation. These study conditions combined with the use of as few exclusion criteria as possible broadened the generalizability of the trial results. In one of the studies, comparing a combination of valproate and lithium with each drug given in monotherapy, patients were methodologically innovatively selected on the tolerability of the combination before randomization (Geddes *et al.*, 2010). This procedure narrowed the generalizability of the trial results to those patients tolerating the combination, but the authors rightly argued that this was a clinically relevant restriction, and even recommended such testing of tolerability in clinical practice before starting a patient on a specific long-term prophylactic agent. Through this enrichment, the likelihood of finding a potential signal was increased, and in fact, despite the use of few exclusion criteria and the simple outcome measures, a signal was found, favoring the combination and lithium over valproate. Interestingly, in the trials comparing lithium with carbamazepine

(Greil *et al.*, 1997; Hartong *et al.*, 2003), lithium was also found to be superior as the overall result. However, in the former of these trials, carbamazepine was superior to lithium in subgroups with atypical features (Kleindienst & Greil, 2000), that is, the generalizability of those results was differential. The trial by Hartong *et al.* (2003) was remarkable in the sense that only patients that were relatively naive regarding prior lithium treatment were included, narrowing the generalizability of study results to a highly relevant clinical subgroup of patients. Besides, it was the only of the investigator-driven trial cited here that was conducted in a double-blind manner. In the trial comparing lithium with lamotrigine, unexpectedly, no overall superiority of lithium was found. This was unexpected since in this comparison, in contrast to the pivotal studies of lamotrigine indicating overall equivalent efficacy between lamotrigine and lithium, lamotrigine was not favored (Licht *et al.*, 2010). The negative results may, at least partly, be related to the ambition to mimic routine clinical conditions as much of possible in interest of generalizability but at the expense of internal validity, for example, by allowing randomization when clinically appropriately even remission had not necessarily been obtained.

Similar to the limitations of results from acute trials in bipolar disorder, results from maintenance trials with a few exceptions generally do not specifically cover the application of drug combinations and the management of patients not responding to first-step treatments. Even though most maintenance trials included patients not responding to various maintenance treatments, no subgroup analyses generalizable to such nonresponders are available. Regarding trials on drug combinations, the study by Geddes *et al.* (2010) is the first three-arm maintenance trial testing a drug combination versus each drug on its own. In the few industry-driven maintenance evaluating drug combinations, the company's drug (an atypical antipsychotic) combined with lithium or valproate was compared with lithium or valproate given alone, but not with the antipsychotic given alone (Tohen *et al.*, 2004; Vieta *et al.*, 2008). Additionally, in these trials, the randomized sample was enriched with patients responding acutely to the combination, thereby narrowing the generalizability of the study results.

In almost all the maintenance trials addressed above, the patients fulfilled the criteria of bipolar disorder, type I. A crucial question is whether the results of these findings can be generalized to patients with bipolar disorder, type II. There is no strict answer to this question, but in the view of the author, it seems reasonable to apply the results of the pivotal studies on lamotrigine to patients with bipolar disorder, type II, who have recurrent episodes of depression. In fact, one trial on lamotrigine in patients with rapid cycling included both patients with bipolar disorder, type I and patients with bipolar disorder, type II (Calabrese *et al.*, 2000). This trial was negative on the primary measure but positive on a secondary measure in the subgroup of bipolar disorder, type II patients. The use of lithium seems also justified in some patients with bipolar disorder, type II based on results from earlier trials (Goodwin & Jamison, 1990).

Regarding the duration of maintenance trials, it can be argued that the 1–2 years' duration of most of the trials is not sufficient to produce results applicable to clinical reality, where patients may be treated for a lifetime. However, in the trial by Licht *et al.* (2010), following a subset of patients up to 5 years, it was clearly demonstrated that all treatment failures essentially took place within the first 1.5 years.

Finally, a comment should be provided to the concern that patients treated outside a trial may have a poorer outcome to a given drug than the same patients would have had if being treated with this drug within the framework of a trial. This concern often relates to the fact that patients within a trial may be provided some support that is not always available in routine settings. However, there is a point often neglected: in most of the maintenance trials discussed here above, the randomized patients are not evaluated beyond the point in time where a treatment emergent point of failure like relapse/recurrence has been decided to take place. In clinical practice. drugs are most often continued beyond emergent symptoms or episodes, based on the experience and observations that prophylactic treatments may require some time to work and accordingly that the amplitude and/or the frequency of episodes may diminish over time (Goodwin & Jamison, 1990). This means that the outcome outside the trial setting in fact may be better than the figures from within the trial may indicate. Trying to reflect this observation, in the trial by Licht *et al.* (2010) treatment emergent events were not recorded until 6 months after randomization.

Supporting the notion here above that some patients treated outside the context of a trial may obtain a better outcome than the overall outcome obtained within a trial, is the approach of narrowing the applicability of trial results of lithium as suggested by Grof (2006). According to this approach, based on observational studies and extensive clinical experience, it is recommended that clinicians carefully select potential excellent lithium responders characterized by, for example, a positive family history and complete interepisodic remission. However, this strategy has yet not been tested in an RCT.

Differential Generalizability or Trial Results Based on Biologic Subgroups in Bipolar Disorder

As outlined in the previous sections, there are very few trial results characterized by a differential generalizability due to a differential treatment response to a given drug in identifiable clinical subgroups of patients within each major indication for drug treatment in bipolar disorder. However, theoretically, there may be a differential generalizability of trial results of any given drug due to differential findings in various biologically different subgroups within each major indication of bipolar disorder. Furthermore, such differential generalizability of trial results may differ from drug to drug, since at least some of the drugs seem to differ in their mode of antibipolar action (e.g., valproate and lithium and atypical antipsychotics).

The assumptions outlined here above may seem reasonable. At least they are underlying the practice of many clinicians when they switch or combine drugs in cases of nonresponse to any first-step treatment, and also underlying the recommendations in many treatment guidelines about management of patients not responding to a first-step treatment (Grunze *et al.*, 2009). Although never proven, such assumptions seem reasonable or at least understandable given the fact that the evidence on how to manage these situations is poor.

SUMMARIZING AND CONCLUDING SECTIONS
Proper Clinical Applicability of Trial Results in Bipolar Disorder: A Brief Guidance

For mania, regardless the informal selection that may characterize the study samples of the positive approval trials, there are consistent and similar results regarding a clinically relevant signal of a pharmacologic effect on mania across all approved drugs given as monotherapy. Even the generalizability in a strict sense is narrowed by the use of formal selection criteria, the broadening of the clinical application of these results to any manic patient seems justifiable and the best evidence-based approach the clinician can choose, regardless severity of illness, comorbid conditions, and clinical circumstances. In addition, it can be justified to broaden the application of the results from the few trials addressing drug combinations to the most severely manic patients and when first-step treatments fail. With the exception of lithium, there is no differential generalizability of the results across the various available treatment options that can give the clinician any guidance in choosing among these options. Therefore, the clinician should be solely guided by safety concerns, patient preference, prior effect, potentials in maintenance phase, and route of administration (Grunze *et al.*, 2009). Compared with the other options, the generalizability of trial results of lithium is a more narrow but well-defined. The well-documented preventive efficacy of lithium adds to the applicability of the results from the mania trials.

For bipolar depression, the trial results are too scarce and scattered to allow any general statements regarding their generalizability. As to quetiapine, despite the generalizability of the results from the pivotal trials is somewhat uncertain, the clinician can probably feel relatively comfortable when he or she applies the results to a relatively broad population of bipolar depressed patients. For lamotrigine and lithium, the conflicting results on efficacy may to some extent be a matter of differential generalizability regarding the various positive and negative results. Finally, for antidepressants, there are still uncertainties regarding generalizability of the existing positive and negative trial results. Taken together, this gives a room for the clinician to apply the results regarding all the various treatment options (Grunze *et al.*, 2010), choosing among them by carefully balancing the same factors as listed above in the context of mania up against each other.

For maintenance treatment, when applying trial results to a clinical situation, the clinician can be guided by the differential generalizability of trial results obtained under various study conditions, for example, pre-randomization enrichment and post-randomization drug discontinuation, in accordance with the way in which the evidence was organized in recently published international guidelines (Grunze *et al.*, 2013). If, for example, a drug chosen for mania is not intended to be continued beyond remission, either because the drug has no proven preventive efficacy or because of emerging side effects, then a drug with proven efficacy under nonenriched conditions, such as lithium, could be added. The differential efficacy of the various drugs including their potential differential pole-specific preventive properties should also be taken into account when applying specific trial results. In addition, besides comparative efficacy, the usual factors of tolerability, prior response or nonresponse, and patient preferences obviously are important when trial results are to be matched to an individual patient. No matter which maintenance treatment is chosen in clinical practice, a strategy of testing long-term tolerability and compliance to the chosen drug during a period before finally deciding for the long-term treatment in order to optimize the treatment effect as developed by the authors of the BALANCE trial seems worth considering (Geddes *et al.*, 2010). When managing emergent insufficient response to any given first-step maintenance treatment, the clinician may beneficially apply combined results from various adequate trials, giving the differential pole specific preventive properties of the various drugs special attention.

From Narrow Generalizability to Broad Applicability: Summarizing the Clinician's Point of View

The clinician is interested in providing a given patient with a given clinical problem a treatment that will work with a likelihood as high as possible. Clearly, it is not a problem for the clinician if the generalizability of results from an RCT is narrow as long as the results, indicating a reasonable effect size, cover the clinical situation that he or she needs to handle. In fact, the best scenario from the clinician's perspective would be if the results from RCTs on the various available treatments had narrow but differential generalizabilities, reflecting that the results of each specific agent had its own specific room for clinical applicability in terms of clinical (or biologic) profile of the patient within each major indication, that is, acute mania, acute bipolar depression, and maintenance phase.

Unfortunately, this is not the scenario with our current level of evidence. Instead, with the exception of lithium for maintenance, the narrowing of generalizability tends to go in the same direction across treatments within each major indication in the sense that it seems to be the same type of selection of study subjects and/or study condition that maximizes the likelihood of response across the treatments. In addition, placebo-controlled trials only extremely rarely can provide a number needed to treat of less than four in bipolar disorder, corresponding to an absolute drug–placebo treatment effect of 25%. The relatively small effect sizes, albeit clinically relevant, calls for strategies to enlarge the effect sizes through narrowing the applicability of trial results to subgroups of potentially excellent responders as has been attempted regarding maintenance treatment with lithium.

When facing clinical reality, the clinician needs to choose between broadening the applicability of given trial results with a relatively narrow generalizability per se, thereby decreasing the likelihood for response in the individual patient or only applying the results to a more narrowly defined group of patients in accordance with the relevant RCT to assure a relatively high likelihood for an individual response. Pragmatically, clinicians may simply apply specific results to an individual patient that is demonstrating the proper diagnosis and treatment phase compatible with the RCT, irrespectively that the patient and the clinical situation may not fully match the study sample and/or study conditions of the RCT. Regarding the latter point, it should be borne in mind that study samples and study conditions are not always clearly described, and at best, there are considerable heterogeneity.

In the management of patients not responding to a first-step treatment, the clinician also needs to deal with the scarcity of trial results specifically generalizable to such situations (e.g., by applying results from different trials into the same situation). A note on dosing should be provided here. Obviously, it makes sense to increase the dose of a given drug in case of nonresponse since patients probably have individual thresholds for response. However, increasing the dose beyond the levels that are used in the relevant trials cannot even be considered a broadening of the applicability of trial results and should generally be avoided.

Through the approach outlined here and by doing his or her best for assuring compliance, managing side effects, providing general support, hope to the patient, or maybe even additional nonpharmacologic therapies, the clinician will practice evidence-based medicine indeed and maximize the likelihood for a favorable outcome in the individual patient.

Approval Trials, Clinical Needs, and Future Perspectives

Overall, as has been described and exemplified in this chapter, the generalizability across all trials in bipolar disorder is often narrow or sometimes uncertain. However, as also outlined, there are ways in which these results reasonably can be applied into the various scenarios of clinical practice. Alternatively, put in another way: even the clinician needs to go beyond the strict generalizability in his or her attempts to match the trial results with a specific patient in a specific clinical situation, this practice can still be considered evidence based.

More specifically, what hopefully has been clarified is that placebo-controlled trials leading to regulatory dug approval as potential proof-of-concept trials of pharmacologic efficacy per se of various agents are in fact a prerequisite for all evidence-based drug treatment. Despite the fact that the generalizability in a strict sense of the results from these trials are generally narrow, and that important clinical situations such as treatment resistance are not covered, these results are valuable starting points in clinical practice and when setting up trials primarily aiming at improving clinical practice. In addition, the three-arm approval trials have provided the field with valuable comparative data and for the maintenance trials in particular provided valuable placebo-controlled data on lithium with a broad generalizability.

A factor adding to the level of applicability of results from the positive approval trials is the relatively favorable profiles regarding adverse effects of many of the drugs introduced since the 1990s.

We still need more efficacious and well-tolerated treatments for bipolar disorder, treatments with novel mechanisms of action that may work with a higher likelihood than the current treatments in smaller, well-defined subgroups of patients. Therefore, approval trials of such potential new treatments are highly welcomed from a clinical point of view. In the meantime, we need to optimize the clinical use of our existing treatment options through conducting trials that move beyond approval and postmarketing purposes. Such trials, typically investigator-driven, may compare various treatments, evaluate combined treatments, or address the management of patients not responding to first-, second-, or third-step treatments.

As has been discussed in this chapter, a broad generalizability is not necessarily better than a narrow. On the contrary, even though trial results with a broad generalizability can be broadly applied, trial results with a narrow applicability may be clinically more useful. Comparative trials based on highly heterogeneous study samples and relatively loosely defined study conditions mimicking clinical routine may contribute only little to clinical practice since no contrasts may be found. Therefore, broadening the selection criteria should be restricted to trials that are so large that it is possible to detect potential signals regarding differential response in subgroups, either clinically or subclinically defined. By broadening the generalizability on one hand through applying a minimum of exclusion criteria and simple study procedures and outcome measures, and maximizing the likelihood of finding a potential signal through selecting patients on compliance on the other hand, the BALANCE trial is an inspiration for future large-scale simple trials (Licht, 2010).

Obviously, in the conduct of trials, funding is a challenge, in particular when industry has no interest in the conduct, which is often the case when the trials do not serve approval or postmarketing purposes. What is needed is therefore large-scale international coordination and collaboration between investigators and optimization of the available independent funding, including local, national, and international sources.

REFERENCES

American Psychiatric Association. (1980). *Diagnostic and statistical manual of mental disorder* (3rd ed.). Washington, DC: American Psychiatric Association.

American Psychiatric Association. (2002). Practice guideline for the treatment of patients with bipolar disorder (revision). *American Journal of Psychiatry, 159*(Suppl. 4), 1–50.

American Psychiatric Association. (2004). *Diagnostic and statistical manual of mental disorder* (4th ed.). Washington, DC: American Psychiatric Association.

American Psychiatric Association. (2013). *Diagnostic and statistical manual of mental disorders* (5th ed.). Washington, DC: American Psychiatric Association.

Bech, P. (1995). *The Bech, Hamilton and Zung scales for mood disorders: Screening and listening.* Berlin: Springer-Verlag.

Berk, M., Dodd, S., Kauer-Sant'anna, M., et al. (2007). Dopamine dysregulation syndrome: Implications for a dopamine hypothesis of bipolar disorder. *Acta Psychiatrica Scandinavica, Supplementum*, 41–49.

Bowden, C. L., Brugger, A. M., Swann, A. C., et al. (1994). Efficacy of divalproex vs lithium and placebo in the treatment of mania. *JAMA*, *271*, 918–924.

Bowden, C. L., Calabrese, J. R., McElroy, S. L., et al. (2000). A randomized, placebo-controlled 12-month trial of divalproex and lithium in treatment of outpatients with bipolar I disorder. Divalproex Maintenance Study Group. *Archives of General Psychiatry*, *57*, 481–489.

Bowden, C. L., Calabrese, J. R., Sachs, G., et al. (2003). A placebo-controlled 18-month trial of lamotrigine and lithium maintenance treatment in recently manic or hypomanic patients with bipolar I disorder. *Archives of General Psychiatry*, *60*, 392–400.

Bowden, C. L., Calabrese, J. R., Wallin, B. A., et al. (1995). Who enters therapeutic trials? Illness characteristics of patients in clinical drug studies of mania. *Psychopharmacology Bulletin*, *31*, 103–109.

Bowden, C. L., Grunze, H., Mullen, J., et al. (2005). A randomized, double-blind, placebo-controlled efficacy and safety study of quetiapine or lithium as monotherapy for mania in bipolar disorder. *Journal of Clinical Psychiatry*, *66*, 111–121.

Bowden, C. L., Mosolov, S., Hranov, L., et al. (2010). Efficacy of valproate versus lithium in mania or mixed mania: A randomized, open 12-week trial. *International Clinical Psychopharmacology*, *25*, 60–67.

Bowden, C. L., Swann, A. C., Calabrese, J. R., et al. (2006). A randomized, placebo-controlled, multicenter study of divalproex sodium extended release in the treatment of acute mania. *Journal of Clinical Psychiatry*, *67*, 1501–1510.

Calabrese, J. R., Bowden, C. L., Sachs, G., et al. (2003). A placebo-controlled 18-month trial of lamotrigine and lithium maintenance treatment in recently depressed patients with bipolar I disorder. *Journal of Clinical Psychiatry*, *64*, 1013–1024.

Calabrese, J. R., Keck, P. E., Jr., et al., Macfadden, W., et al. (2005). A randomized, double-blind, placebo-controlled trial of quetiapine in the treatment of bipolar I or II depression. *American Journal of Psychiatry*, *162*, 1351–1360.

Calabrese, J. R., Suppes, T., Bowden, C. L., et al. (2000). A double-blind, placebo-controlled, prophylaxis study of lamotrigine in rapid-cycling bipolar disorder. Lamictal 614 Study Group. *Journal of Clinical Psychiatry*, *61*, 841–850.

Calabrese, J. R., Vieta, E., El-Mallakh, R., et al. (2004). Mood state at study entry as predictor of the polarity of relapse in bipolar disorder. *Biological Psychiatry*, *56*, 957–963.

Cipriani, A., & Geddes, J. R. (2009). What is a randomised controlled trial? *Epidemiologia e Psichiatria Sociale*, *18*, 191–194.

Colom, F., Vieta, E., Daban, C., et al. (2006). Clinical and therapeutic implications of predominant polarity in bipolar disorder. *Journal of Affective Disorders*, *93*, 13–17.

Cook, R. J., & Sackett, D. L. (1995). The number needed to treat: A clinically useful measure of treatment effect. *BMJ*, *310*, 452–454.

Elwood, J. M. (1988). Selection of subjects for study. In J. M. Elwood (Ed.), *Causal relationships in medicine* (pp. 38–57). Oxford: Oxford University Press.

Frank, E., Prien, R. F., Jarrett, R. B., et al. (1991). Conceptualization and rationale for consensus definitions of terms in major depressive disorder. Remission, recovery, relapse, and recurrence. *Archives of General Psychiatry*, *48*, 851–855.

Geddes, J. R. (2005). Large simple trials in psychiatry: Providing reliable answers to important clinical questions. *Epidemiologia e Psichiatria Sociale*, *14*, 122–126.

Geddes, J. R., Calabrese, J. R., & Goodwin, G. M. (2009). Lamotrigine for treatment of bipolar depression: Independent meta-analysis and meta-regression of individual patient data from five randomised trials. *British Journal of Psychiatry*, *194*, 4–9.

Geddes, J. R., & Carney, S. (2009). Evidence-based medicine and neurophysiology. *Clinical EEG and Neuroscience*, *40*, 59–61.

Geddes, J. R., Goodwin, G. M., Rendell, J., et al. (2010). Lithium plus valproate combination therapy versus monotherapy for relapse prevention in bipolar I disorder (BALANCE): A randomised open-label trial. *Lancet*, *375*, 385–395.

Geddes, J. R., & Harrison, P. J. (1997). Closing the gap between research and practice. *British Journal of Psychiatry*, *171*, 220–225.

Geller, B., Cooper, T. B., Sun, K., et al. (1998). Double-blind and placebo-controlled study of lithium for adolescent bipolar disorders with secondary substance dependency. *Journal of the American Academy of Child and Adolescent Psychiatry*, *37*, 171–178.

Goldstein, B. I., Sassi, R., & Diler, R. S. (2012). Pharmacologic treatment of bipolar disorder in children and adolescents. *Child and Adolescent Psychiatric Clinics of North America*, *21*, 911–939.

Goodwin, F. K., & Jamison, K. R. (1990). *Manic-depressive illness*. New York: Oxford University Press.

Goodwin, G. M., Bowden, C. L., Calabrese, J. R., et al. (2004). A pooled analysis of 2 placebo-controlled 18-month trials of lamotrigine and lithium maintenance in bipolar I disorder. *Journal of Clinical Psychiatry*, *65*, 432–441.

Greil, W., Ludwig-Mayerhofer, W., Erazo, N., et al. (1997). Lithium versus carbamazepine in the maintenance treatment of bipolar disorders – a randomised study. *Journal of Affective Disorders*, *43*, 151–161.

Greil, W., Ludwig-Mayerhofer, W., Steller, B., et al. (1993). The recruitment process for a multicenter study on the long-term prophylactic treatment of affective disorders. *Journal of Affective Disorders*, *28*, 257–265.

Grof, P. (2006). Responders to long-term lithium treatment. In M. Bauer, P. Grof, & B. Müller-Oerlinghausen (Eds.), *Lithium in neuropsychiatry. The comprehensive guide* (pp. 157–178). Abingdon: Informa Helathcare.

Grof, P., Akhter, M. I., Campbell, M., et al. (1993). *Clinical evaluation of psychotropic drugs for psychiatric disorders. Principles and proposed guidelines* (Vol. 2). Seattle: Hogrefe & Huber Publishers.

Grunze, H., Vieta, E., Goodwin, G. M., et al. (2009). The World Federation of Societies of Biological Psychiatry (WFSBP) guidelines for the biological treatment of bipolar disorders: Update 2009 on the treatment of acute mania. *World Journal of Biological Psychiatry*, *10*, 85–116.

Grunze, H., Vieta, E., Goodwin, G. M., et al. (2010). The World Federation of Societies of Biological Psychiatry (WFSBP) guidelines for the biological treatment of bipolar disorders: Update 2010 on the treatment of acute bipolar depression. *World Journal of Biological Psychiatry*, *11*, 81–109.

Grunze, H., Vieta, E., Goodwin, G. M., et al. (2013). The World Federation of Societies of Biological Psychiatry (WFSBP) guidelines for the biological treatment of bipolar disorders: Update 2012 on the long-term treatment of bipolar disorder. *World Journal of Biological Psychiatry*, *14*, 154–219.

Hartong, E. G., Moleman, P., Hoogduin, C. A., et al. (2003). Prophylactic efficacy of lithium versus carbamazepine in treatment-naive bipolar patients. *Journal of Clinical Psychiatry*, *64*, 144–151.

Houston, J. P., Tohen, M., Degenhardt, E. K., et al. (2009). Olanzapine-divalproex combination versus divalproex monotherapy in the treatment of bipolar mixed episodes: A double-blind, placebo-controlled study. *Journal of Clinical Psychiatry*, *70*, 1540–1547.

Kleindienst, N., & Greil, W. (2000). Differential efficacy of lithium and carbamazepine in the prophylaxis of bipolar disorder: Results of the MAP study. *Neuropsychobiology*, *42*(Suppl. 1), 2–10.

Koukopoulos, A., & Ghaemi, S. N. (2009). The primacy of mania: A reconsideration of mood disorders. *European Psychiatry*, *24*, 125–134.

Larsen, J. K., Porsdal, V., Aarre, T. F., et al. (2009). Mania in the Nordic countries: Patients and treatment in the acute phase of the EMBLEM study. *Nordic Journal of Psychiatry*, *63*, 285–291.

Licht, R. W. (1998). Drug treatment of mania: A critical review. *Acta Psychiatrica Scandinivica*, *97*, 387–397.

Licht, R. W. (2001). Limitations in randomised controlled trials evaluating drug effects in mania. *European Archives of Psychiatry and Clinical Neuroscience*, *251*(Suppl. 2), II66–II71.

Licht, R. W. (2006). Lithium in the treatment of mania. In M. Bauer, P. Grof, & B. Müller-Oerlinghausen (Eds.), *Lithium in neuropsychiatry. The comprehensive guide* (pp. 59–72). Abingdon: Informa Helathcare.

Licht, R. W. (2010). A new BALANCE in bipolar I disorder. *Lancet*, *375*, 350–352.

Licht, R. W. (2012). Lithium: Still a major option in the management of bipolar disorder. *CNS Neuroscience & Therapeutics, 18*, 219–226.

Licht, R. W. (2013). Is it possible to evaluate true prophylactic efficacy of antidepressants in severely ill patients with recurrent depression? Lessons from a placebo-controlled trial. The fifth trial of the Danish University Antidepressant Group (DUAG-5). *Journal of Affective Disorders, 148*, 286–290.

Licht, R. W., & Bech, P. (2009). How to manage mania not responding to a first-step 2 weeks treatment with quetiapine – a report from a prematurely discontinued randomised clinical trial. *Acta Psychiatrica Scandinavica, 120*, 334–335.

Licht, R. W., Bysted, M., & Christensen, H. (2001). ICD-10 versus DSM-IV diagnostic criteria for bipolar mania: A clinical comparison. *Bipolar Disorders, 3*(Suppl. 1), 19–20.

Licht, R. W., Gijsman, H., Nolen, W. A., et al. (2008). Are antidepressants safe in the treatment of bipolar depression? A critical evaluation of their potential risk to induce switch into mania or cycle acceleration. *Acta Psychiatrica Scandinavica, 118*, 337–346.

Licht, R. W., Gouliaev, G., Vestergaard, P., et al. (1994). Treatment of manic episodes in Scandinavia: The use of neuroleptic drugs in a clinical routine setting. *Journal of Affective Diseases, 32*, 179–185.

Licht, R. W., Gouliaev, G., Vestergaard, P., et al. (1997). Generalisability of results from randomised drug trials. A trial on antimanic treatment. *British Journal Psychiatry, 170*, 264–267.

Licht, R. W., Nielsen, J. N., Gram, L. F., et al. (2010). Lamotrigine versus lithium as maintenance treatment in bipolar I disorder: An open randomized effectiveness study mimicking clinical practice. The 6th trial of the Danish University Antidepressant Group (DUAG-6). *Bipolar Disorders, 12*, 483–493.

McElroy, S. L., Bowden, C. L., Collins, M. A., et al. (2008). Relationship of open acute mania treatment to blinded maintenance outcome in bipolar I disorder. *Journal of Affective Disorders, 107*, 127–133.

McIntyre, R. S., & Wong, R. (2012). Asenapine: A synthesis of efficacy data in bipolar mania and schizophrenia. *Clinical Schizophrenia & Related Psychoses, 5*, 217–220.

Mendez, M. F. (2000). Mania in neurologic disorders. *Current Psychiatry Reports, 2*, 440–445.

Moller, H. J., Grunze, H., & Broich, K. (2006). Do recent efficacy data on the drug treatment of acute bipolar depression support the position that drugs other than antidepressants are the treatment of choice? A conceptual review. *European Archives of Psychiatry and Clinical Neurosciences, 256*, 1–16.

Muller-Oerlinghausen, B., Retzow, A., Henn, F. A., et al. (2000). Valproate as an adjunct to neuroleptic medication for the treatment of acute episodes of mania: A prospective, randomized, double-blind, placebo-controlled, multicenter study. European Valproate Mania Study Group. *Journal of Clinical Psychopharmacology, 20*, 195–203.

Nielsen, J., Kane, J. M., & Correll, C. U. (2012). Real-world effectiveness of clozapine in patients with bipolar disorder: Results from a 2-year mirror-image study. *Bipolar Disorders, 14*, 863–869.

Niufan, G., Tohen, M., Qiuqing, A., et al. (2008). Olanzapine versus lithium in the acute treatment of bipolar mania: A double-blind, randomized, controlled trial. *Journal of Affective Disorders, 105*, 101–108.

Pacchiarotti, I., Bond, D. J., Baldessarini, R. J., et al. (2013). The International Society for Bipolar Disorders (ISBD) Task Force report on antidepressant use in bipolar disorders. *American Journal of Psychiatry, 170*(11), 1249–1262.

Pope, H. G., Jr., McElroy, S. L., Keck, P. E., Jr., et al. (1991). Valproate in the treatment of acute mania. *Archives of General Psychiatry, 48*, 62–68.

Prien, R. F., Caffey, E. M., Jr., & Klett, C. J. (1972). Comparison of lithium carbonate and chlorpromazine in the treatment of mania. Report of the Veterans Administration and National Institute of Mental Health Collaborative Study Group. *Archives of General Psychiatry, 26*, 146–153.

Rothman, K. J. (1986). *Modern epidemiology*. Boston: Little, Brown and Company.

Sachs, G. S., Nierenberg, A. A., Calabrese, J. R., et al. (2007). Effectiveness of adjunctive antidepressant treatment for bipolar depression. *New England Journal of Medicine, 356*, 1711–1722.

Sackett, D. L. (2011). Explanatory and pragmatic clinical trials: A primer and application to a recent asthma trial. *Polskie Archiwum Medycyny Wewnętrznej, 121*, 259–263.

Schatzberg, A. F., Blier, P., Delgado, P. L., et al. (2006). Antidepressant discontinuation syndrome: Consensus panel recommendations for clinical management and additional research. *Journal of Clinical Psychiatry, 67*(Suppl. 4), 27–30.

Schene, A. H., Wijngaarden, B. V., & Baaren-Marcelis, J. W. V. (1994). Randomization and generalization in psychiatric research. *International Journal of Methods in Psychiatric Research, 4*, 1–5.

Smith, L. A., Cornelius, V., Warnock, A., et al. (2007). Acute bipolar mania: A systematic review and meta-analysis of co-therapy vs. monotherapy. *Acta Psychiatrica Scandinavica, 115*, 12–20.

Storosum, J. G., Fouwels, A., Gispen-de Wied, C. C., et al. (2004). How real are patients in placebo-controlled studies of acute manic episode? *European Neuropsychopharmacology, 14*, 319–323.

Swann, A. C., Bowden, C. L., Calabrese, J. R., et al. (2002). Pattern of response to divalproex, lithium, or placebo in four naturalistic subtypes of mania. *Neuropsychopharmacology, 26*, 530–536.

Thase, M. E., Macfadden, W., Weisler, R. H., et al. (2006). Efficacy of quetiapine monotherapy in bipolar I and II depression: A double-blind, placebo-controlled study (the BOLDER II study). *Journal of Clinical Psychopharmacology, 26*, 600–609.

Tohen, M., Chengappa, K. N., Suppes, T., et al. (2002). Efficacy of olanzapine in combination with valproate or lithium in the treatment of mania in patients partially nonresponsive to valproate or lithium monotherapy. *Archives of General Psychiatry, 59*, 62–69.

Tohen, M., Chengappa, K. N., Suppes, T., et al. (2004). Relapse prevention in bipolar I disorder: 18-month comparison of olanzapine plus mood stabiliser v. mood stabiliser alone. *British Journal of Psychiatry, 184*, 337–345.

Tohen, M., Greil, W., Calabrese, J. R., et al. (2005). Olanzapine versus lithium in the maintenance treatment of bipolar disorder: A 12-month, randomized, double-blind, controlled clinical trial. *American Journal of Psychiatry, 162*, 1281–1290.

Tohen, M., Sanger, T. M., McElroy, S. L., et al. (1999). Olanzapine versus placebo in the treatment of acute mania. Olanzapine HGEH Study Group. *American Journal of Psychiatry, 156*, 702–709.

Tohen, M., Vieta, E., Calabrese, J., et al. (2003). Efficacy of olanzapine and olanzapine–fluoxetine combination in the treatment of bipolar I depression. *Archives of General Psychiatry, 60*, 1079–1088.

Tsapakis, E. M., Soldani, F., Tondo, L., et al. (2008). Efficacy of antidepressants in juvenile depression: Meta-analysis. *British Journal of Psychiatry, 193*, 10–17.

Vaidyanathan, U., Patrick, C. J., & Iacono, W. G. (2012). Examining the overlap between bipolar disorder, nonaffective psychosis, and common mental disorders using latent class analysis. *Psychopathology, 45*, 361–365.

van der Loos, M. L., Mulder, P. G., Hartong, E. G., et al. (2009). Efficacy and safety of lamotrigine as add-on treatment to lithium in bipolar depression: A multicenter, double-blind, placebo-controlled trial. *Journal of Clinical Psychiatry, 70*, 223–231.

Vieta, E. (2005). The treatment of mixed states and the risk of switching to depression. *European Psychiatry, 20*, 96–100.

Vieta, E., & Cruz, N. (2012). Head to head comparisons as an alternative to placebo-controlled trials. *European Neuropsychopharmacology, 22*, 800–803.

Vieta, E., Montgomery, S., Sulaiman, A. H., et al. (2012). A randomized, double-blind, placebo-controlled trial to assess prevention of mood episodes with risperidone long-acting injectable in patients with bipolar I disorder. *European Neuropsychopharmacology, 22*, 825–835.

Vieta, E., Suppes, T., Eggens, I., et al. (2008). Efficacy and safety of quetiapine in combination with lithium or divalproex for maintenance of patients with bipolar I disorder (International Trial 126). *Journal of Affective Disorders, 109*, 251–263.

Weisler, R. H., Nolen, W. A., Neijber, A., et al. (2011). Continuation of quetiapine versus switching to placebo or lithium for maintenance treatment of bipolar I disorder (Trial 144: A randomized controlled study). *Journal of Clinical Psychiatry, 72*, 1452–1464.

Wijkstra, J., Schubart, C. D., & Nolen, W. A. (2009). Treatment of unipolar psychotic depression: The use of evidence in practice guidelines. *World Journal of Biological Psychiatry, 10*, 409–415.

World Health Organization. (1992). The ICD-10 classification of mental and behavioral disorders: *Clinical desciptions and diagnostic guidelines.* Geneva: World Health Organization.

Yildiz, A., Guleryuz, S., Ankerst, D. P., et al. (2008). Protein kinase C inhibition in the treatment of mania: A double-blind, placebo-controlled trial of tamoxifen. *Archives of General Psychiatry, 65*, 255–263.

Yildiz, A., Vieta, E., Leucht, S., et al. (2011). Efficacy of antimanic treatments: Meta-analysis of randomized, controlled trials. *Neuropsychopharmacology, 36*, 375–389.

Young, A. H., McElroy, S. L., Bauer, M., et al. (2010a). A double-blind, placebo-controlled study of quetiapine and lithium monotherapy in adults in the acute phase of bipolar depression (EMBOLDEN I). *Journal of Clinical Psychiatry, 71*, 150–162.

Young, A. H., McElroy, S. L., Olausson, B., et al. (2014). A randomised, placebo-controlled 52-week trial of continued quetiapine treatment in recently depressed patients with bipolar I and bipolar II disorder. *World Journal of Biological Psychiatry, 15*, 96–112.

Young, R. C., Schulberg, H. C., Gildengers, A. G., et al. (2010b). Conceptual and methodological issues in designing a randomized, controlled treatment trial for geriatric bipolar disorder: GERI-BD. *Bipolar Disorders, 12*, 56–67.

Chapter Eleven

Clinical Trials in Developing Countries: Challenges in Design, Execution, and Regulation

Chittaranjan Andrade[1] and Tim Appaiah[2]

[1]*National Institute of Mental Health and Neurosciences, Bangalore, India;*
[2]*ClinPrax Research Pvt Ltd, Bangalore, India*

CHAPTER OUTLINE

INTRODUCTION

More than two decades have passed since clinical trials went global; that is, when pharmaceutical majors began conducting regulatory trials in many centers at the same time, spread across countries and continents. This chapter discusses circumstances that make conducting clinical trials in developing countries different from those in the developed world; India is selected as a case in point. The presentation is narrative and is based on experience; there are few-to-no data on country-specific demographics, or nationally

Clinical Trial Design Challenges in Mood Disorders. DOI: http://dx.doi.org/10.1016/B978-0-12-405170-6.00011-7

representative epidemiologic studies of any nature, let alone those conducted with the assistance of standardized diagnostic interviews.

Since the 2000s, there has been a virtual genesis of the clinical trial industry in India (Yee, 2012). Courses are now offered that train participants in the fundamentals of clinical research and site monitoring. Clinical research organizations have been launched. Clinical sites that specialize in conducting industry-driven clinical trials have sprung up. These developments have resulted from the interest shown by multinational pharmaceutical companies in conducting Phase III clinical trials in the country. Frost and Sullivan estimated that in 2010–2011 the Indian clinical trial industry was worth US$450 million (Editorial, 2013). What led to these developments, and why; and what are the plus and minus points of these developments? These matters are briefly examined in the sections that follow.

CLINICAL TRIALS IN DEVELOPING COUNTRIES: WHO GAINS, AND WHY?

Who gains when pharmaceutical companies conduct their clinical trials in developing countries such as India? First and most important, science gains because it is probably easier to separate signal from noise in the analysis of data from developing countries (Andrade, 2013). There are many reasons for this. Patients with major mental illness in India are less likely to have comorbid psychiatric conditions, including concurrent alcohol and substance abuse, and less likely to have personality disorders. Thus, the treated sample is diagnostically cleaner. In addition, patients in India have strong family support: most families ensure medication adherence, bring patients for follow-up, and take over the responsibilities of the affected member until he or she recovers. Thus, protocol adherence and study retention rates are high, decreasing the last-observation-carried-forward problems that compromise the validity of a study.

Most patients have medical leave and can return to work after they recover; many employers, in fact, even allow patients diminished responsibilities until such a time that they regain full functional status. Thus, study retention rates are high for both inpatient and outpatient protocols. The high levels of family and social support also makes it less likely that patients will be treatment-refractory for reasons related to environmental stress.

Pharmaceutical companies gain because they obtain cleaner and more reliable results when the science is good. There are other, more practical gains, too, for the industry. Developing countries are overpopulated and there is pressure on the healthcare system to cater to the needs of mentally ill people. Therefore, recruitment targets are more quickly met. Salaries, costs of living, and clinical trial expenses are lower, and so trials can be completed on lower budgets. Patients tend to accept a paternalistic model of healthcare, and so dropout rates are low. An added advantage in countries such as India is that almost all investigators are fluent in English, the medium in which protocols are drafted and instruction is provided.

For the investigators who conduct the clinical trials gain, some of the gain is financial, because remuneration from the pharmaceutical industry is far greater than that obtained from patients and salaries. For self-employed investigators, the financial gain is personal. For those working in institutions, the moneys are paid to the employers, but these monies can often be deployed for the investigator's independent research, or to improve the facilities available in the department; and occasionally, to supplement their own salary income.

Some of the gain is academic, because investigators are trained in good clinical practice and in research processes. This empowers them to design and conduct their own studies, should they want to do so. Some of the gain is more mundane – site investigators get to travel, meet other investigators from other countries, and enjoy the prestige of being part of a large research consortium.

For the patients who are subjects in the clinical trials gain, healthcare in developing countries is seldom high in quality, and when free care is unavailable, many patients find it hard to afford the necessary investigations and medicines. When they participate in clinical trials, patients receive high-quality, individualized inpatient or outpatient care at no cost; in fact, even their travel and food expenses for visits are reimbursed.

Lastly, society gains, because when clinical trials are conducted in developing countries, locally relevant pharmacodynamic and pharmacokinetic data are generated, and regulatory approval for later marketing in these countries is more easily obtained on the strength of the data collected. This is, of course, also an advantage for the industry.

CLINICAL TRIALS IN DEVELOPING COUNTRIES: WHO LOSES, AND WHY?

There are downsides to completing clinical trials in developing countries. In their everyday responsibilities, site investigators are commonly burdened by understaffing and high patient loads, and few patients in routine clinical care receive more than 10 minutes of attention per visit. Clinical trials magnify the burden because each enrolled patient requires at least 1–2 hours per visit. This is a particular problem when an investigator has several clinical trials (sometimes, a dozen or more) running simultaneously (Yee, 2012). Therefore, principal investigators hire junior staff as subinvestigators specifically for the execution of research protocols. When principal investigators delegate responsibilities so that they can continue to attend to their regular responsibilities, it defeats the purpose of having a senior investigator in charge of the research. Furthermore, the subinvestigators realize that their employment is temporary and they have no scope for advancement, and so seek better employment opportunities. If subinvestigators resign during the course of the trial, recruitment is compromised until new staff are appointed and trained. Changing research staff results in changing quality of assessment, and introduces background noise that masks the quality of the signal (Andrade, 2013).

Insufficient experience, motivation, supervision, and time are issues that can result in poorer quality control and greater intersite variation in results;

science is compromised, and the trials may fail for reasons that are unrelated to the efficacy of the treatment under study.

When English is not the native language of most of the patients, the informed consent forms and some of the rating instruments may need to be translated into the many local languages. Usually, only forward and back translation exercises are conducted to establish superficial validity of the translation; the psychometric properties of the translated instruments are not established.

In this regard, interactive voice response protocols can be particularly problematic. The automated interview will need to be conducted in the patient's native language, the dialects and accents of which can vary widely from district to district. Patients from rural backgrounds, especially those who are illiterate or elderly, often find it difficult to first understand what is being asked and next have the presence of mind to press an appropriate button on the telephone. Some site investigators address this problem by setting the phone on speaker mode and assisting the patient with the buttons; but this defeats the purpose of the exercise.

There are other practical problems, too. For example, not all patients understand the importance of punctuality of follow-up, and some may come outside the window defined for a scheduled visit. Likewise, not all patients understand the importance of strict adherence to the protocol; they may take disallowed medications, fail to come fasting for a scheduled visit, or make other mistakes.

Besides science and the pharmaceutical industry, patients can also lose when clinical trials are conducted in developing countries. There is, of course, no assurance that patients will receive the trial drug or that the trial drug will be effective. Patients know that even if the medication is effective, they will no longer receive it after the study is over. All these are acknowledged risks. The hidden risk is that patients will be exploited. Exploitation may start at recruitment when uneducated, illiterate patients believe that their doctors are acting in their best interests and therefore consent to participate in the clinical trial without understanding the contents of the informed consent form and without understanding the associated risks. Issues related to consent in India were discussed by Chaturvedi (2007). One solution for this problem is to add a one-page summary to the detailed consent form, and to have a list of questions that the patient is expected to answer correctly to ensure comprehension of the contents of the form. This approach was adopted in an Indian trial by D'Souza et al. (2013). Another solution is to require the patient to take the form home and discuss his or her participation with relatives and friends before signing the consent form. However, such approaches are innovative and voluntary rather than made compulsory by regulation.

Exploitation may continue when patients are allowed or even encouraged to remain in the trial despite failure to respond to treatment. Exploitation is at its worst when patients experience an adverse event that requires intervention, investigation, or even hospitalization; such is not always provided free of cost because these expenses are not part of the clinical trial budget. Indeed, the patient is covered by insurance, but from where would a poor patient obtain the money to pay the hospital until the insurance company admits, allows, and reimburses the claim? How would an illiterate patient even fill in an insurance claim? Moreover, given that the insurance company is located in a far away developed country, how will the patients pursue their claims or even sue for justice if they are denied their dues? Some of these issues were discussed by Rao and Andrade (2013).

Some ethics committees in India have addressed this concern by insisting on local insurance (Rao & Andrade, 2013). However, local insurance companies can be as intransigent as international ones when it comes to honoring claims. Unfortunately, life in developing countries is little valued; it is common for the maximum sum insured, payable on the event of death, to be as little as in the region of US$1500.

A small but sometimes significant concern is that blood is assigned considerable psychological significance in some societies, and so every occasion of blood drawing can be traumatic to some patients, especially when the quantity drawn exceeds 5 mL.

Lastly, patients, science, and society lose when the trial drug fails to separate from placebo and the trial is left unpublished. Patients who participated in order to further the cause of science and society are cheated because nobody learns about the negative outcomes. The loss to science and society is obvious (Rao & Andrade, 2013).

THE REGULATORY ENVIRONMENT

The regulatory environment is of concern in developing countries because there is no assurance that it is adequate for the local needs. At a central level, governmental clearances are required; in India, this is usually effected at the offices of the Drug Controller General of India. Central clearance is plagued by bureaucratic delays.

At the site level, clearances are issued by a local ethics committee, the composition and functioning of which are governed by regulations; in India, the document detailing these regulations is titled *Schedule Y*. This document is a part of the *Drugs and Cosmetics Act, 1940 and Rules, 1945 of India* and is available online. Whereas institutions can constitute their own ethics committees, until recently self-employed investigators relied on independent ethics committees; that is, freelancing bodies that oversaw research activity for a fee. New regulations require all ethics committees to be approved and registered by the offices of the Drug Controller General of India.

It is common for ethics committees to meet infrequently, such as once in 3 months, and for the review to address only recruitment numbers, progress in the trial, and occurrence of adverse events, if any. Detailed audits of trials are almost never conducted. Thus, there is no assurance that all ethical concerns will always be adequately addressed.

Special Issues

There are often country-specific regulatory issues. For example, in India, Phase I clinical trials are generally not allowed unless the drug has been developed in the country (Srinivasan, 2013). If Phase I data are available from other countries for a drug that was developed outside India, then a Phase I trial may be allowed inside India (Central Drugs Standard Control Organization, 2011). Biologic samples cannot be exported such as for pharmacogenetic tests unless special clearances have been obtained.

DISCUSSION: DEVELOPMENTS IN INDIA

This section addresses ethical and regulatory developments in India during 2011–2014. In 2012, the Drug Controller General of India responded to a right-to-information enquiry with the news that deaths during clinical trials numbered 288, 637, 668, and 438 during 2008, 2009, 2010, and 2011, respectively; some of these could have been due to the medications whereas others could have been due to the illness (e.g., cancer) for which the medications were being trialed. However, compensation was paid in only 22 cases (Anon, 2012).

There was little subsequent improvement. For example, in March 2013, the Union Health Minister, Government of India, informed Parliament that of 2868 deaths that had occurred during clinical trials from 2005 to 2012, only 89 had been attributed directly to the trials, and compensation had been paid in only 45 of these cases. These payments were small; for example, Novartis paid only about US$5000 for one trial-related death (Editorial, 2013). Strong concern has been expressed in the lay press that these figures for trial-related deaths are underestimates (Srinivasan, 2013). Ethical concerns were strongly expressed not only in the lay press (Datta, 2013) but also in medical journals with worldwide coverage (Sugarman et al., 2013; Yee, 2012), although specific allegations were robustly refuted by site investigators (Pauranik et al., 2012).

Concerns about the manner in which clinical trials were being conducted, and especially concerns about deaths that had occurred, resulted in a Supreme Court-directed cessation of regulatory approval for the conduct of clinical trials in the country. In late 2013, the Supreme Court of India at last permitted five pending trials that had been approved by the Drug Controller General of India, requiring that the informed consent process be audiovisually recorded. A further 157 trials were placed on hold, pending evaluation by a Technical and Apex Committee with regard to the following parameters (Anon, 2013):
1. assessment of risk versus benefit to patients;
2. innovation vis-a-vis existing therapeutic options;
3. medical needs of the country.

Data from the Central Drugs Standard Control Organization showed that new drug clinical trial approvals dropped from 264 in 2008 to 98 in 2011. In 2013, fewer than 10 new drug trials were approved. This regulatory holdup has resulted in clinical trials by pharmaceutical majors such as Alembic, Lupin, Cadilla, Sun Pharma, and Biocon leaving the country, and in some clinical trial facilities closing down (Das & Balakrishnan, 2014). Some of the regulatory changes proposed or implemented are considered overreactions or unduly restrictive (Shukla, 2013; Sugarman et al., 2013). Thus, from being a favored destination for clinical trials, as before (Yee, 2012), India has now become a destination to avoid. The story is India is still evolving, with several more developments expected.

CONCLUDING NOTES

This chapter has been written with industry-driven clinical trials in mind. However, the contents are equally applicable to investigator-initiated clinical trials.

It is likely that what has been described here in the context of Indian experience is past history for many developed countries, and the future for many developing countries. It is hoped that as societies evolve, investigators, industry, and the regulatory environment will all learn from the mistakes committed and benefit from the solutions found so that clinical trials can be executed efficiently without compromising scientific and ethical standards.

REFERENCES

Andrade, C. (2013). Signal-to-noise ratio, variability, and their relevance in clinical trials. *Journal of Clinical Psychiatry*, *74*, 479–481.

Anon. (2012). *Drug trials claim over 2,000 lives in four years*. <http://www.thehindu.com/sci-tech/health/policy-and-issues/drug-trials-claim-over-2000-lives-in-four-years/article3589099.ece/> Accessed 04.08.14.

Anon. (2013) SC *allows 5 clinical trials, sets new rules for consent*. <http://www.deccanherald.com/content/364472/sc-allows-5-clinical-trials.html/> Accessed 04.08.14.

Central Drugs Standard Control Organization. (2011). *Draft guidance on approval of clinical trials & new drugs*. <http://www.cdsco.nic.in/writereaddata/Guidance%20for%20New%20Drug%20Approval%2023.07.2011.pdf/> Accessed 04.08.14.

Chaturvedi, S. (2007). A review of Indian publications on ethical issues regarding capacity, informed consent, and placebo controlled trials. *Internet Journal of Mental Health*, *5*(2) <http://ispub.com/IJMH/5/2/7089/> Accessed 04.08.14.

D'Souza, D. C., Radhakrishnan, R., Perry, E., et al. (2013). Feasibility, safety, and efficacy of the combination of D-serine and computerized cognitive retraining in schizophrenia: An international collaborative pilot study. *Neuropsychopharmacology*, *38*, 492–503.

Das, S., Balakrishnan, R. (2014). *Clinical trials and tribulations at home push companies abroad*. <http://www.business-standard.com/article/companies/clinical-trials-and-tribulations-at-home-push-companies-abroad-114012401033_1.html/> Accessed 08.08.14.

Datta, A. (2013). *Trial errors*. <http://www.thehindubusinessline.com/industry-and-economy/trial-errors/article5231671.ece/> Accessed 04.08.14.

Editorial. (2013). *Clinical errors: Clinical trials need better regulation*. <http://www.business-standard.com/article/opinion/clinical-errors-113102700673_1.html/> Accessed 04.08.14.

Pauranik, A., Bharani, A., Bhargava, S., et al. (2012). Misleading report on clinical trials in India. *Lancet*, *379*, 1947–1948.

Rao, T. S., & Andrade, C. (2013). Ethical issues in psychiatry research: Special concerns for India. *Indian Journal of Psychiatry*, *55*, 1–2.

Shukla, S. (2013). India's amended trials regulations spark research exodus. *Lancet*, *382*, 845.

Srinivasan, S. (2013). *When clinical trials become dangerous*. <http://www.thehindubusinessline.com/opinion/when-clinical-trials-become-dangerous/article5237461.ece/> Accessed 04.08.14.

Sugarman, J., Bhan, A., Bollinger, R., et al. (2013). India's new policy to protect research participants. *British Medical Journal*, *347*, f4841.

Yee, A. (2012). Regulation failing to keep up with India's trials boom. *Lancet*, *379*, 397–398.

Index

Note: Page numbers followed by "*f*" and "*t*" refer to figures and tables, respectively.